GENTLECARE

Changing the Experience of
Alzheimer's Disease
in a Positive Way

GENTLECARE™

Changing the Experience of Alzheimer's Disease in a Positive Way

M O Y R A   J O N E S

Hartley & Marks
PUBLISHERS

Published by

HARTLEY & MARKS PUBLISHERS INC.

P.O. Box 147   3661 West Broadway
Point Roberts, WA   Vancouver, BC
98281   V6R 2B8

GENTLECARE is the registered trademark of
Moyra Jones Resources Ltd.

LIBRARY OF CONGRESS CATALOGING-IN-PUBLICATION DATA
Jones, Moyra, 1936-
    Gentlecare: Changing the Experience of Alzheimer's Disease /
Moyra Jones.
        p.   cm.
    Includes index.
    ISBN 0-88179-171-7
        1. Alzheimer's disease—Patients—Care.   2. Alzheimer's disease—
Patients—Rehabilitation.   3. Alzheimer's disease—Patients—Family
relationships.   4. Alzheimer's disease—Patients—Home care.
    I. Title.
RC523.J66   1998
362.1'96831—dc21   98-26019
                                                           CIP

Set in SCALA and SCALA SANS by The Typeworks
Cover design by Diane McIntosh
Printed in the U.S.A.

This one is for Rob,
who is always there
when it matters

GENTLECARE™

In geology, a discontinuity is a break in the ordered layering of the earth's strata, often caused by the tectonic forces which bend the strata until it breaks. We know these breaks as earthquakes.

Alzheimer's disease is not unlike the tectonic forces which cause earthquakes. Alzheimer's disease strips away the humanity of those afflicted by the disease, layer by layer. It exhorts from family caregivers a level of involvement beyond their ability to provide, and it causes major and minor seismic events within healthcare systems which are poorly prepared to manage the crisis.

The Gentlecare Lifecare Prosthetic System (Gentlecare™) offers support in living to the individual suffering from the disease, and knowledge, skills, and support for family and professional care providers.

There is an old Chinese saying:

A butterfly flaps its wings
Once and the air all over
The earth is changed forever

Gentlecare has adopted the butterfly as its logo in an effort to depict the gentle and complex approach advocated in the care of people with dementing illnesses.

Each one of us, in whatever our role, who helps recall a memory, restores dignity, or rights a wrong for any of these vulnerable people, changes the world forever in ways we may never know.

I appreciate your company on this journey of exploration, challenge, and success. I can be contacted at:

Moyra Jones Resources Ltd.
8264 Burnlake Drive
Burnaby, British Columbia V5A 3K9
Canada

Phone: 604-421-1680
Fax: 604-421-1753
E-Mail: jonesb@direct.ca
Website: www.Gentlecare.com

...dream, believe, experience

Contents

Acknowledgments

No book is the result of the author's efforts alone. So my grateful acknowledgment is offered to many people who have given of their time, energy, expertise, experiences, and suggestions.

I want to thank:

The families and victims of Alzheimer's disease who welcomed me into their lives and courageously shared their stories. They are true heroes.

My two men: Robert, who never faltered in his belief that this book was possible; and Marc, my son and soul mate, who spent more hours at the computer, and made more cups of tea, than I care to remember.

Joyce Wright, whose love and support gives new meaning to the word friendship.

Lorna Seaman, for her generous contributions to my understanding of nutrition, and the joy she brought to our creative endeavors.

My former colleague Alix McGinity, for her support and editorial comments on the subject of assessment.

Sandy Telford, an outstanding Gentlecare practitioner, who bravely tested my ideas and generously shared her experiences.

John Piacitelli, a unique and precious advocate for elderly people, who believed in Gentlecare, and urged me to write about it.

Olga Greenwell, who encourages me through good times and bad, and always comes up with the right word.

The professional care providers who work each and every day "in the trenches" and who understand the challenges of providing Alzheimer's care.

My dear friends Michael J. and Hardtimes Morgan who unfailingly kept me company through every hour of writing.

I shall always be grateful to Douglas Gray, who with great generosity of spirit went out of his way to provide me with wise counsel.

Every author should be lucky in their choice of publishing house. I am very grateful to the people at Hartley & Marks for their caring, persistence, and spirit; to my publisher Vic Marks who believed in this book; to Susan Berlin, my lion-hearted editor who helped move my ideas to a different level; to managing editor Susan Juby, for awesome support in the final stages; indeed all the fine people who contributed to bringing this book into being.

The hundreds and hundreds of people who have taken the time to write to me with ideas, anecdotes, stories, butterflies, and good wishes.

This book would not have been possible without everyone's love.

—Moyra
Ajijic, Mexico
February 1999

Foreword

The biggest disease today is not leprosy or tuberculosis,
but rather the feeling of being unwanted.
—Mother Theresa, *Observer,* 3 October 1971

The prevalence of Alzheimer's disease in the older population is a tragedy unmatched in any other age group. This tragedy is compounded by the type of care they frequently receive when placed in long-term care facilities.

Moyra Jones was faced with this situation when her father and other family members fell victim to the disease. Based on this personal experience and her own professional expertise, she dedicated herself to developing a system of care that expresses her conviction that dementia does not rob an individual of his or her individuality. In Moyra's Gentlecare system for dementia care, the caregiver is required to treat the person with dementia as a unique human being with the same need for respect, recognition, and self-worth as a person without dementia.

Her philosophical approach emphasizes the need for everyone involved in the care of the impaired person, regardless of function or job description, to accept and value the dignity and worth of the impaired person. Caregivers are further expected to contribute to the creation of a prosthetic environment free of physical restraint that provides the person with dementia the support needed to make up for the progressive loss of functions resulting from the illness.

The benefits of the Gentlecare system have been felt not only by people with Alzheimer's disease, but by fellow residents, family members, and staff as well.

In this book, Moyra shares her philosophy on which her care system is based, and provides much-needed practical guidelines for families and other caregivers to use in their care of people with dementia, and in their relationships with one another. Whether you are a caregiver or not, this book will challenge you to examine your beliefs and feelings about being old, and about having dementia or some other mental illness. You will be asked to look at your attitudes, your expectations, and the behaviors you encourage and reinforce in the older people you serve.

By so doing, you will gain the satisfaction of knowing that you have encouraged in them the discovery of new meaning and purpose in their lives, without a feeling of being unwanted, regardless of their age or mental status.

—John D. Piacitelli, MSW, MPH
Mental Health Program Administrator
Elderly Services, Washington State
Mental Health Division
Tacoma, WA, USA

Alzheimer's disease is a progressive disease that we cannot really change, nor can we avoid its ultimate outcome. The disease is frightening for professionals and relatives because we cannot stop its destructive effects.

Among both professional and lay caregivers, some think that Alzheimer's disease is incurable, that the afflicted person cannot be helped, and that custodial care is the only kind of care possible. Others believe that people with Alzheimer's can be rehabilitated if they are involved in intensive activities to improve their mental and physical capacities. In reality, however, inappropriate activities compromise afflicted people and often trigger aggressive reactions.

I had difficulties caring for people with Alzheimer's disease, and doubts about the possibility of improving the level of care in my facility. Then I was introduced to Moyra and Gentlecare. I experienced a paradigm shift, and am now an enthusiastic supporter of the need for special care for dementia victims based on the Gentlecare prosthetic model.

My thinking changed because of the evidence put before me. Alzheimer's disease is incurable—but the Alzheimer patient is not untreatable! Gentlecare provides an alternative to patient neglect or the traditional, and unreachable, rehabilitation goal of functional improvement. Gentlecare is based on a prosthetic model aimed at maximizing the well-being of Alzheimer patients by using a three-pronged program: adapted environments, personal contact, and supportive activities. We, doctors and families, could not accept the unhappy conclusion that there was nothing we could do. For us, Gentlecare is a new and powerful alternative. In her book, Moyra explains how these three elements elevate the quality of care for Alzheimer patients.

The main surprise for the reader will be the book's rich and detailed review of the everyday life of people with Alzheimer's, their families, and caregivers. *Gentlecare* offers many useful suggestions on every aspect of daily routine, from nutrition to sleep patterns. But for me, the best part is the new mind-set and the new approach to people with Alzheimer's that one gets from reading Moyra's book: build new supportive environments, find new solutions for behavioral problems, imagine new ways of improving well-being, and you will succeed in taking care of them. Every person is an individual, and caring for people is not simply a matter of applying a formula, but rather of recognizing each individual's uniqueness. That, I think, is the main lesson to be learned from this book, from Gentlecare, from Moyra Jones.

—Antonio Guaita, MD
Medical Director
Instituto Geriatrico, Camillo Golgi,
Abbiategrasso (Milano), Italy

Prologue

This book began a long time ago. My family and I became caught up in caring for my father in the 1960s, long before Alzheimer's disease became a household word. No one in our circle of acquaintances had ever heard of Alzheimer's. There were no books, no journals, no articles, and no health services available to help us sort through the complex problems that confronted us. I was told the disease was rare, non-hereditary, that it affected only memory. I was told, in fact, that it did not exist!

My mother was encouraged to stay at home in the small village where she and my father had always lived and to call the church if she needed help with my father. We soon learned that no one wanted to be involved in my father's health problems. The physicians encouraged rest and a change of pace, and finally, massive doses of anti-psychotic medication, which left my father rigid and as brain-dead as a zombie. There was "no room at the inn" in any health care facility. Even years later I can vividly remember every detail of our journeys through the corridors of emergency services, acute medical/surgical wards, and palliative care units. There were brief sojourns in the empty rooms of pediatric departments, and finally four years of moves to and fro within extended care units.

I remember going to visit my father in hospital one day in the beginning, when he still knew where he was and what was happening to him. He was stretched flat on his back with a double layer of sheeting wrapped around him from his chin to his toes, pinning him to the bed. His face was blue. He was making pitiful choking sounds like a small trapped animal. I remember my frantic search for scissors, and the paralyzing anxiety that

My father and me.

hampered me as I cut the sheets that bound him. I can still feel his breath on my face when he finally responded to my resuscitation efforts. And I will never forget his eyes looking at me and asking, "Why?"

What had happened to the health care system that I had worked in since I was 13 years old? How could the organizations I had later studied and worked within be failing my father when he needed them most? Why were some people receiving superb health care and treatment at the same time that my father was being treated like a leper by the very same system?

Why? Why? Why? These same questions are still being asked by families today.

Later on, when my father's Alzheimer's disease had progressed, I learned that the problems we had encountered in the beginning were just the tip of the iceberg. Things got worse, much worse. Sometimes in my ignorance and despair I thought I had done my father a disservice by rescuing him from asphyxiation.

And today, in hindsight and the light of knowledge cast by our growing understanding of Alzheimer's, I think, "If only I had known then what I know now!"

*My mother and father enjoyed
a unique relationship.*

My father was a gentle, caring man who adored his wife, his daughter, and his dogs. He had a fine sense of community, believing that each of us had a bounden duty to extend our own good fortune to those less fortunate in our community. I have lovely images of him at dusk in our backyard, leaning on the pump as he talked to a farmer about money to buy some needed equipment, or counseled some young couple on ways to manage the purchase of a home.

He was a naturalist who practiced conservation long before it became the popular thing to do. He adored roaming outdoors on foot or by canoe. His love of space, freedom, and movement became his deadly enemies later in his dance with dementia. He loved people, animals, plants, jobs, projects, emergencies, challenges, music, fun, teasing, travel, his church, his home, his garden, and especially butter tarts!

My dad was a fine problem solver. He would consider a problem for days, trying various strategies or approaches until he found a solution that was just right. As a little girl I remember watching in fascination as he built stone walls. He selected each stone with great care, seeing colors and images in the stone that my untrained eye could not see. Sometimes he would abruptly turn the stone completely upside down and find the perfect fit. Then he would grin at me, drawing me into a lovely feeling of satisfaction.

As Alzheimer's disease invaded his mind, my father followed these same lifelong patterns—touching, moving, fitting, taking apart, stacking, tearing, turning things upside down, until he had the whole house in one awful mess. For the most part my mother and I followed him, trying to restore order and get him to sit down and be quiet!

My dad was a wonderful gardener, so I was aghast the day he began to dig holes in his beautiful lawn. At first I tried to entice him into the house, the car, anywhere, just so long as I could keep him from ruining the lawn. Then suddenly I realized what was happening: he was working! This man was engaged in a job, and not about to be distracted from it by my protestations. Where once he had created wonderful flower beds, now he dug holes. It was hard for me to regard the destructive act of digging holes in the same way I viewed gardening, but given the nature of the disease consuming his mind, this activity was the best version of his former skills that he could manage: digging holes equaled gardening.

This insight was infinitely liberating for me. It allowed me to understand his concentration and persistence. It helped me to see life through his eyes. It took me behind the disease, and gave me back my father.

And so I encouraged him to dig holes—and I filled them in. We spent endless joyful hours at this activity. Once I was able to look beyond the specific activity, I was able to appreciate and even enjoy this limited, distorted version of his former skills.

I was able to laugh with him and celebrate our shared accomplishments. We could stop for a tea break, clean up together, and go into the house with that tired glow that only gardening can give.

Years later, as my father sat restrained in a chair, my heart broke as I sensed his frustration and despair. Where could I find the words to explain to hospital staff that he wanted to dig holes, to have a job, to be free, to feel again a sense of accomplishment and self-worth? Within the hospital setting there was no possibility of an old man digging holes. When he tried, he was given medication and restrained in a wheelchair.

And so we lost him—not so much to the disease, but rather to the system. He was in the wrong place, with the wrong disease, at the wrong time.

I remember going to visit him each evening after work, untying his restraint, helping him find his balance, and then trying to keep up with him as he raced down the corridors and out into the fresh air. My father was an outdoors man: strong, active, utterly tireless. It must have been sheer hell for him to sit confined for days on end, not permitted to stand or move about. I can remember a staff member saying to me as we passed by, "Is that Len? I didn't know he could walk!" But how could she? She had only seen him in a wheelchair. She was a part of the system that fed, changed, and tidied patients, gave them their medications, and focused on urgent matters. She was one of an insufficient number of people doing endless tasks in a limited amount of time. How could she be expected to know my father? And how could I, knowing her work routine, say to her: "Please, he needs to be digging holes"?

So what was this physically strong man, with no need of medical treatment, doing in the middle of a facility designed to treat and manage physical illness? Talk about square pegs in round holes! No wonder he couldn't fit in. No wonder everyone was at their wits' end in trying to "cope" with him.

Most staff I talked to didn't really understand my father's illness. When I explained some of his behaviors in terms of his disease process, they would say, "Oh, that makes sense! That's why he does so-and-so!" And I would think how hard it must be to care for people in such an intimate way without knowing who they were or why they acted the way they did.

It took my father a long time to die. Some days I could not find him in the fog of drugs and dementia. And some days he was with me in an eerie fashion that made me think, "Oh my God! He's still here. He still feels. He knows." One night, in preparing him for sleep, I adjusted the restraint jacket that held him flat on his back on the bed. And he looked straight at me and said, "Why are you doing this to me?"

Why, indeed? I had no answer for him then.

Somewhere in the system of which he was a part, it had been decided that this physically well man would now be tied to a bed on his back for hours and hours during the night. Sometimes he would lie in his own waste, sometimes he would shout and swear. Always he would tear at the restraint, pleading for release or crying, "Why are you doing this to me?" Those words, and his image, burn in my brain even to this day.

I believe there is a better way.

Throughout my father's illness, significant people emerged for him. His grandson Marc who visited and chatted a blue streak with him, a homemaker who had a knack for making him laugh, a nurse from Hong Kong who forged an unlikely and lasting bond with him. And I, as only daughter, connected with him in ways that changed both our lives. But it was my mother who mattered most. She was his touchstone, his security. She tried to be with him all the time because when she was, he was content. When he was upset, it was she who could calm him. He would do anything she asked. Even when he could no longer utter her name, he would smile, or whistle, or on some occasions touch her hand.

At the time, none of us really appreciated the drain of my father's illness on my mother. Fixated as we were on the horror of my father's unfolding disease, we neglected to notice her physical and emotional exhaustion. We failed to identify her overwhelming grief at the loss of her life partner. Because he was alive, we never addressed the losses we were all feeling until it was much too late, and my mother, too, was tragically ill. Today, medical journals abound with articles on caregiver burnout. But careful study is required before we truly understand the complexity of the caregiving relationship throughout the continuum of the disease.

Though surrounded by me and wonderfully caring staff, my father waited until my mother was at his side before he died. How could this be when the disease destroys all cognition? I don't know—I only know it happened. In those few moments I learned how powerful and enduring the familial relationship really is, and what a potent, irreplaceable therapeutic force it can be.

A few years ago, I was privileged to help one of my mother's old friends at the time of her death. She laughed and said, "Oh honey! I can hardly wait to see your mother and father tonight. [They had both predeceased her.] I'm going to tell them what you are doing and all the progress that's been made with your dad's disease." I remember marveling at a faith so strong and comforting.

Two friends to the very end.

Sometimes in the quiet, I imagine these three old friends observing all the positive efforts being made to change the way we care for people experiencing dementing illness and their family members. I imagine my father's delight when he sees old men in Gentlecare units moving furniture, piling wood, even digging holes! And it surely would please my mother to see caregivers taking care of themselves, gaining the knowledge and skills they need to do the job of caregiving, and also attending to their grieving, and to a life after dementia.

A lot has changed in 30 years—but much remains the same. This book is about Gentlecare: a system designed to make changes.

PART ONE

UNDERSTANDING ALZHEIMER'S DISEASE

UNDERSTANDING ALZHEIMER'S DISEASE

ASSESSMENT IN DEMENTIA CARE

A NEW APPROACH TO PROGRAMS

NUTRITION IN DEMENTIA CARE

DESIGN FOR LIVING

PEOPLE AND THEIR IMPACT ON CARE

GENTLECARE
The Prosthetic Life Care System for People with Dementia

1

Old Problems, New Issues

If only, when one heard
That Old Age was coming,
One could bolt the door,
Answer "not at home!"
And refuse to meet him!
— Old Chinese drinking song

It has been said that societies are judged by the way they treat their very old and their very young. Old age is a fact of life. All of us have fathers, mothers, husbands, wives, lovers, and friends who have lived beyond mid-life. By the year 2000, one-fifth of our population will be 65 years of age or older. Most of those people—70 percent of them—will be active, wise, strong, and dynamic, living independently in their communities, and enjoying life fully. However, increasing numbers of elderly people are not aging in accordance with conventional expectations.

Older people are becoming the principal client group for all health care services, acute and chronic care alike. And 10 to 12 percent of those elders 65 years and older requiring any kind of health care services will do so because of a dementing illness. As the average age of the population rises, the number of people so afflicted will increase dramatically, until nearly half of all people over 85 will suffer from some form of progressive dementia—most often Alzheimer's disease. For every one of these unfortunate people, at least one family member and often more will be involved in providing care.

People with dementia deeply disturb our ideas about old age and how it should unfold. The eccentricities of the cognitively alert can be looked upon as charming quirks. Those same behaviors in dementia sufferers are judged as further evidence of their incompetence. Cognitively impaired elders—perhaps our parents—defy our expectations. For many grown children, the notion of a parent being less than "parent-like" is unthinkable. People with dementia don't fit the mold of "normal aging." More importantly, they don't fit into our existing health care system. For people with dementing illness, there is no refuge—not in their own homes, their communities, or within our social service and health care systems. Consequently, they are overwhelmed by fear and anxiety; they are deprived of normal roles and relationships, surrounded by a conspiracy of silence, and unable to affect the outcome of events in their own lives.

Many theories of disease assign to the luckless ill the ultimate responsibility both for falling ill and for getting well.

—SUSAN SONTANG,
*ILLNESS AS A
METAPHOR*

DEMENTIA

Dementia refers to over 70 diseases that cause a grouping of symptoms which results in progressive deterioration of brain cells, particularly those responsible for memory and thought. The cause is often unknown, and therefore a cure is currently unavailable. Dementing illness results in dysfunction in all aspects of daily living and interpersonal relationships. This category of diseases often was referred to as senility.

People with dementia are oppressed by the recognition that they are a problem to their families and to others—a situation they are helpless to alter. At the most vulnerable time in their lives they are often abandoned by the very systems they have counted on and contributed to all their lives: their families, their churches, and their health care systems.

An estimated 70 percent of all care given to persons with dementia is provided by elderly women, who are often ill themselves and certainly exhausted. Their ability to advocate on behalf of impaired family members is questionable. Trained in the importance of maintaining dignity and surviving through resignation and fortitude, older women often don't make waves. Because current health care practices fail to meet the needs of people with dementia, 80 percent of caretakers

choose instead simply to care for their family members at home, often
at a tragic cost to their own health.

As dementing illnesses like Alzheimer's disease spread more
widely, the advocacy torch is being passed to a younger, more vocal
group of caregivers: daughters and daughters-in-law who make up the
fastest-growing group of new caregivers. Younger family members trying to come to grips with the problem of dementia are less willing to
settle for inadequate health care for their family members. The challenge for those of us on the front line is to focus our anger and find a
better—a different—way to meet the needs of people with dementia
and their families.

Alzheimer's disease exists in two forms: *early onset disease,* which
normally shows its first signs between the ages of 45 and 60; and *late
onset disease,* which can become evident at any time after the age of 60.
Both types of the disease are on the increase.

As yet, the cause of the increase in early onset Alzheimer's (or pre-
senile dementia of the Alzheimer's type) is unknown. The increase in
the late onset form of the disease *(senile dementia)* is probably explained
in part by the fact that people are simply living longer. As well, it is
known that about 10 to 15 percent of people with Alzheimer's come
from families in which significant numbers of people have had the disease; this is known as Familial Alzheimer's disease.

In his Global Deterioration Scale, Dr. Barry Reisberg suggests that
Alzheimer's disease parallels *in reverse* the developmental stages of
childhood. As a child gains developmental mastery over his life, so a
person experiencing dementia declines through the same stages, losing control over the various aspects of life. As people live through the
process of Alzheimer's disease, it is possible to correlate their functional levels with those of children at similar stages. For example, by
the time a person with Alzheimer's requires 24-hour supervision, he
or she is probably operating at the *developmental* level of a child of seven
or eight while being seventy-three years old chronologically. Such a
person is not a child, but rather childlike in terms of the ability to manage life tasks and need for appropriate supports.

It's worth noting that, as a rule, when children become ill our health

Nothing she did or said was quite what she meant but still her life could be called a monument shaped in a slant of available light and set to the movement of possible music.

—JUDITH DOWNING,
"THE GRAND-
MOTHER CYCLE"
CONVERSE QUARTERLY

care system goes to exquisite lengths to prepare them for hospitalization, to allay their fears, to develop an environment that helps them get well and does not frighten them, and to ensure that a family support system is place. But when an elderly man with dementia becomes so dysfunctional that he requires round-the-clock supervision, his admission to hospital is often very different. Not infrequently, he is transported to hospital in an emergency vehicle or a stranger's car. He is placed in a communal living situation, surrounded by large numbers of people he doesn't know. Often it is suggested that his spouse or other family member leave, "until he settles in," which in some cases can be for a period of several weeks. He is shown to a bedroom, directed to a dining room, and then expected to manage in a strange and complex environment that may resound with telephones, intercoms, emergency buzzers, and alarm systems. There is not a familiar face in sight.

The person has no idea what is happening to his family, his pets, his house, or any of the responsibilities he may feel he has. Even if he is reassured on these matters, the disease causes him to forget the information as soon as he hears it. Fear and anxiety are the natural result, and often medication is administered to calm or quiet him. Medication creates even more confusion and disorientation, and so the fear and anxiety escalate.

It is curious that the health care system responds so very differently to people from two generations with very similar needs. On the one hand, the child is cherished and supported; on the other hand, the older person is treated with insensitivity and disregarded.

Although it is often painful, even unacceptable, for us to regard our elders with dementia as childlike, awareness of Alzheimer's reverse development process helps us to understand their vulnerability and need for special support. Furthermore, since we have gone through exactly the same stages of development that people with dementia traverse in reverse, we can recall how it feels to be helpless, afraid, to have one's opinions discounted, and be unable to make decisions independently. Those of us who have supported children through their developmental stages have already had the experience of how to give just the right amount of help, and how to withdraw support as they develop confidence and skills. This experience is invaluable in caring for people with dementia—if only caregivers learn to use it in reverse.

With such awareness, we can see how unreasonable we have been in our expectations of these frightened, vulnerable old people. We begin to see that they really require life care—not medical care—as their disease inevitably progresses. We begin to understand the pain and dilemma of family caregivers, and their power to help family members.

> *Evil thrives on apathy*
> *and cannot exist*
> *without it.*
>
> —HANNAS ARENDT

All we have learned about special, age-appropriate environments can help us design comfortable and comforting accommodation for older people with dementing illnesses. By using existing resources from families, communities, and the health care system, we can devise care strategies and support systems that truly and humanely meet the needs of these people.

It is no longer appropriate to regard elderly people as a homogeneous group who require the same type of environment, the same health care strategies, and the same solutions for dealing with their life problems. Whether they are "young-old" or "old-old," "young-old" with physical problems or "old-old" with cognitive problems, "over-all old" or simply aging "problem-old," our elders deserve appropriate responses and care from individuals, social structures, institutions, and communities.

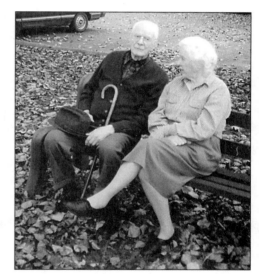

The provision of appropriate services to the elderly requires a new commitment on the part of society at all levels. It is not so much a question of right or wrong, but rather a determination to do things differently.

Changes in the Older Population

Aging is everyone's tomorrow. It may be that one of us is beginning to experience the challenge of changes in health, status, or role that accompany older age. Or perhaps in mid-life we find ourselves caught up in the lives of our parents or grandparents. For many of us who work in

TYPICAL BREAKDOWN
OF ELDERS IN
HEALTH CARE FACILITIES

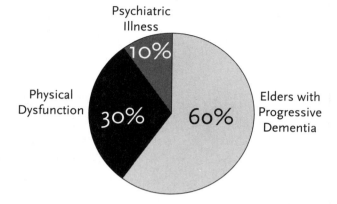

FIGURE 1-1

health care services, older people are becoming our principal client group, whether we provide acute or chronic care.

In the past, the health care problems of older people were generally seen as complex physical illnesses associated with aging. Today older people with physical illnesses are living longer, responding to ever-expanding medical and technological strategies, and asking to live in their own homes or in alternative arrangements within their communities. Older people with exclusively physical illnesses now form a minority group in chronic care, total care, or palliative care institutions. Elders who suffer from psychiatric disorders other than dementia now also form a minority in the health care system, as large psychiatric institutions downsize and send mentally ill people back to their local communities. These people are referred to as "psychogeriatrics," a pejorative term applied only to older people who experience psychiatric illness. (Children are never referred to as "psychopaediatrics!")

A disturbing proportion of older people in our communities, however, are elders experiencing some type of dementia or cognitive impairment. They are ultimately referred to our health systems for care. Older people with dementias may comprise up to 60 to 70 percent of all elders who use health care services.

For example, two out of three older people who use emergency services may have a dementing illness in addition to other health problems. Acute care medical facilities care for significant numbers of older people with dementia who require medical or surgical services, or who are awaiting placement in long-term care facilities. And three-quarters of the people who live in intermediate long-term care facilities have a dementing illness alone or in combination with other illnesses.

Chronic care, extended care, or total care facilities provide services for those who are greatly at risk of developing, or who already have, primary dementias. The challenge of providing appropriate care for these people is compounded by the fact that any of these conditions may exist together with other illnesses. For instance, it is not uncommon to find someone with Alzheimer's disease who is profoundly depressed, or someone with Parkinson's disease who also has cardiac dysfunction.

Furthermore, each of these people has at least one caregiver, often elderly as well, who is very likely to be exhausted and ill. By the year 2000, providing gerontological care for the elderly will be as challenging and complex as delivering acute medical care.

Forces That Shape the Care We Give

As people live longer, more of them develop some of the diseases of aging. Since the causes of many of these diseases remain obscure, effective treatment is elusive, and in some cases impossible. The traditional ways of caring for elderly people are proving inadequate and even inappropriate for the "new" types of illness and dysfunction we are encountering.

Suddenly, health services that were designed for other purposes are faced with providing residential and personal care to growing numbers of cognitively impaired mid-life and elderly persons—as well as providing advice and support to their family caregivers. The focus is shifting from health care to life care.

The challenge of the next decade is to evolve a new way of thinking about health and disease. The dehumanization of health care becomes especially critical when we consider services for older people. We need to re-conceptualize the way we think of illness. We can no longer think of it as just a physical condition that can be cured, or at least managed. If illness includes limited cognitive abilities, as it more frequently does among older people, we need to consider how to best preserve the whole person, and support a lifestyle that is meaningful and whole-some.

Is it reasonable to believe that structures and systems designed to ameliorate physical illness will work effectively for persons who are cognitively impaired, but relatively fit physically?

Troubling questions follow from this, and raise deep clinical and ethical problems—problems that quick-fix approaches won't solve. To achieve the necessary changes within health care systems requires that we change our perceptions regarding old age, and most especially, our view of progressive dementing illness and mental illness in the elderly. The services and practices we offer people with cognitive impairment and their families must be based on new and current knowledge, combined with effective management practices. Having recognized that most of the old paradigms, structures, and beliefs about caring for people with dementias were based on an incomplete understanding of their real needs, we must learn to approach problems differently. If people with dementia don't respond to the type of care we offer, then we have to change the type of care we give.

Is it reasonable, for example, to expect an elderly person experiencing dysfunction due to brain cell death to be able to live comfortably within existing health care facilities? Is it even possible?

I MET AN ELDERLY MAN AT HIS HOME, *and we walked in his garden. He pointed with delight to various trees that were his favorites. His family was seeking assistance in choosing a facility because his wife was ill and could no longer manage his care on her own.*

Three months later, I visited him in an institution, where he sat in a geriatric chair (a chair with a lock-down tray used for restraint purposes). When he saw me he began to cry, and said, "I am imprisoned in this machine. Please, please set me free!" When we did release him from the restraint, it was evident that he could no longer walk. His legs and ankles were swollen and his knees and hips had lost their range of movement. He had been changed into a "total care" patient by the system—not by the disease.

The North American approach to care of the elderly employs a *biomedical model* of care—a perspective that focuses on pathology and interventions that relieve symptoms or cure disease. This emphasis defines and shapes the systems we create, and the attitudes and behaviors we experience within the system.

In this model, people become "patients" and "patients" become their disease—"the gallbladder in room 203." The spectacular success of new technology and medical practices has overshadowed the harm that such highly technological and disease-specific systems can cause.

The reliance on the biomedical model to explain the experience of dementing illness has resulted in the medicalization of dementia. We have attempted to control dementia with medication, which can actually exacerbate problems if improperly used.

Can professional and lay personnel, without appropriate education or understanding of clinical issues, be expected to meet the challenges of Alzheimer's care?

The biomedical approach overlooks the social construction of dementia, in terms of changes in a person's functional deterioration, and the subsequent dynamics of caregiving relationships and community roles. The model also fails to take into account the impact of treatment contexts and environmental pressures on both the person with dementia and caregivers.

A place to live one's life to the fullest.

Viewing dementia as a medical problem that must be "fixed" has led us to focus on managing the problem behaviors that result

Not a place to wait for life's end.

CHAPTER
ONE

from brain dysfunction. Consequently, problem behavior has come to be seen as an inevitable part of dementing illness, when in fact this need not be the case. For example, wandering, which has come to be seen as a pivotal aspect of Alzheimer's disease (Does he wander or not? Does he wander into someone else's room? Does he wander at night? Outdoors?), is not part of the clinical definition of Alzheimer's disease. Do we discuss causes? No. Instead, we are preoccupied with wandering! And wandering may be a function of being afraid, lonely, disoriented, anxious, or just going about one's business. Wandering may be simply explained as thirst, the need to find a bathroom, or boredom. Thus, behavior not considered abnormal if displayed by others is often judged harshly if exhibited by someone known to be cognitively impaired. Who among us has not wandered through a mall, or a mountain meadow, or the ancient part of a city?

Is it reasonable to expect that elderly family caregivers—on their own—can meet the needs of persons devastated by dementia on a 24-hour basis for years and years?

The biomedical view of dementia is narrow, limited, and distorted in that it disregards the social forces that affect the progression of dementia. For example, we expect older people with dementia to live communally with other elders who may be cognitively alert, or who may suffer from psychiatric disorders. At this most vulnerable time of their lives, people with dementia are expected to adapt to and comply with living situations that people without dementia would find daunting. The psycho-social experience of dementing illness simply cannot fully be addressed within the confines of biomedical concepts.

For example, if a person with dementia exhibits problematic behavior, harmful to others or herself, she is eligible for admission to a Special Care Dementia Unit (SCU). Once admitted, if the stress-free environment together with support offered by knowledgeable staff results in the person no longer displaying "violent" or problematic behavior, then she is no longer eligible to remain in the specialized environment. She is regarded as being "cured" of difficult behavior, and no longer in need of dementia care. It is not unusual to see such people transferred back to exactly the same situation that first caused the problem. And it is very common to see this tragic cycle played out again and again during the course of the disease.

CHARACTERISTICS OF THE ACUTE BIOMEDICAL CARE PARADIGM

- The biomedical model of treatment is preoccupied with the treatment of symptoms and signs of disease and cures.
- Primary interventions are invasive strategies such as medication and surgery.
- Staff are encouraged to be emotionally neutral.
- The body and mind are regarded as separate entities.
- Environments are institutional in nature and technologically intensive.
- Patient dependency and compliance with medical treatment is encouraged.
- The health care professional is the authority and custodian of pertinent information and solutions.
- Labor is divided along professional or territorial lines.
- The emphasis is on efficiency.

Aging is not a disease— it's a lifelong process that's very individual.

—MARY FEDNIK

FIGURE 1-2

Attitudes and Malignant Myths that Shape the Way We React

Ageism

Ageism is discrimination on the basis of age. Older persons are often rendered invisible in life, in literature, and in films, or stereotyped as decrepit, lonely, or mean-spirited members of society who have little or nothing to contribute. Older persons are denied their individuality or often allowed only a very narrow spectrum of activities or acceptable behaviors.

Ageism can also be the social construction of aging. Rather than viewing aging as a normal process, we see it in terms of disease and dysfunction. This shapes the way we think and talk about old age, and the way we design health care systems. Biases are often so ingrained that we fail to recognize or identify our prejudices.

A YOUNG DOCTOR *who supervised an emergency department in a large hospital told me he felt older persons with dementia "use up far too much of our available health care resources. Do you really expect me to treat an old man with dementia rather than a child, or before I attend to a younger person? Honestly, Moyra, I don't know why you bother!"*

Commonly, older persons really get no health care treatment at all. What they get is more like health care "management." In many countries, there are health care workers called "case managers" who are responsible for developing health care plans for elders assigned to them—whether they agree to be "managed" or not. Nowhere is the management of elders more obvious than in the way we deal with older people with cognitive impairment. When we apply attitudes, language, and actions informed by ageism to management of the elderly, we produce dysfunction and loss of quality of life at an alarming rate.

Therapeutic Nihilism

The treatment of disease in older people, particularly the treatment of dementing illness, is plagued by *therapeutic nihilism:* the belief that nothing can be done to arrest the inevitable decline of intellectual and self-care abilities. It is true that no medical protocol currently exists to treat or cure progressive dementing illness. This does not mean, however, that nothing can be done to help people live through the process of dementia, or to help their families provide effective support. Therapeutic personal care, if appropriately applied, can dissipate problem behavior and assist the person with dementia to enjoy a relatively decent quality of life.

Infantilization

Let's get the potty line over with.

—ONE CARE AIDE
TO ANOTHER

Being old in some cultures still carries with it the notion of respect. However, in our North American culture, status-giving roles and functions for the elderly are being destroyed, without satisfactory replacements. Tragically, many elderly people have accepted the negative social attitude about aging. One such attitude, *infantilization* of the elderly, is systemic in our health care programs. It can be defined as providing care activities for an elderly person beyond what is required by the person's needs or capacities. Infantilization results in learned helplessness. A vicious cycle is established whereby patronizing the elderly reduces their self-esteem, causing them to want to do less for themselves, which in turn makes them more helpless and childlike, and more in need of help.

Health care personnel, especially, are in a strategic position to affect the self-image of the institutionalized elderly. The negative attitudes and expectations of staff are frequently conveyed to elderly people, resulting in institutionally induced dependency. Troubling examples include the increasing numbers of elderly persons who are fed by staff or pushed about in wheelchairs, even though they are able to feed or walk by themselves. A classic example of infantilization is the children's high chair, modified for use by adults—the geriatric chair with the lock-down tabletop. It is a common restraint measure.

Losing people before they die is one of the most stressful aspects of dementia.

—NANCY MACE,
THE 36-HOUR DAY

Much more obvious and poignant examples are to be found in the experience of older persons with dementing illnesses. As they grow progressively more dependent, and their capacity for adaptation diminishes, they are regarded as persons who have lost their "adultness." As they begin to act like children in their helplessness, power is transferred to health care personnel. With a dismaying disregard for the remaining potential of afflicted people, they are:

- excluded from decision-making about their care;
- patronized;
- fed, dressed, bathed, and put to bed, although capable of performing many of these functions independently; and
- reprimanded and subjected to other forms of punishment when behavior deviates from the norms of the institution.

I REMEMBER VIVIDLY *a conversation with an old gentleman who was participating in a summer respite vacation for Alzheimer caregivers and their afflicted family members. I had been advised by the man's professional caregiver that he always went to bed directly after supper. When I offered to show him to his room, he became very reluctant and upset, so I asked him what was bothering him. He said, "I am a person! I want to stay up with the other people. Why do I have to go to bed?" When I encouraged him, by all means, to join us in front of the fireplace, he reached in his pocket and produced a mouth organ, with which he entertained us for several hours.*

Along with many other social, cultural, and moral issues, the myths of ageism and the models of care we use create serious problems for older people when they seek help from the existing health care system. And the cultural framework of the health care system limits and distorts the work of health care providers, including medical personnel, architects, interior designers, and people using the system.

One must wait until the evening to see how splendid the day has been.

—SOPHOCLES

Let's remember that the longer we live, the more we know; and the more we know, the more beautiful we are. We can actively create a new context for the experience of aging by shifting the outlook towards older people in our society. We are a cold and uncaring culture in our treatment of [North] Americans. In China, elders are respected and revered, which is a large part of why the Chinese live so long as healthy and productive citizens. We have thought that youth is better, and "thinking makes it so." Not because it is an objective truth, but only because it is a thought we carry and manifest in our collective experience.

—MARIANNE WILLIAMSON,
RETURN TO LOVE

2

Models are Maps
for Action

*A model or paradigm is the set of ideas
that serves as a blueprint
or pattern for action.*

Older adults clearly need health care provided in a different way. To design more appropriate services, health care providers must first ask, "Why do we do things the way we presently do them?" Unless we examine the ideas that govern our actions—past and present—we are doomed to live with systems in the future that serve neither older people who need care, their families, nor professional care providers. Health care providers will continue to waste their creative energy on crisis management, finding Band-Aid solutions and never addressing the real problems, never asking older people themselves how they would like help to make their lives more fulfilling.

To generate ideas and guide our thinking in finding solutions we need new models. A model is a device we can use to find our way in the practice of care. We need to dust off our maps! This chapter examines the various models health care providers presently use to deliver care to people with dementing illness. So often, health care providers are driven not by the needs of people but by a sense of urgency. We just want to do something to fix the situation. We want to get the work done. We need to meet a deadline. We feel pressure to comply with rules, standards, schedules. We busy ourselves with paperwork or non-productive tasks. As a result, we frequently find ourselves working without any model or map. Perhaps worse, we may find that we are all using different maps. The work we do becomes fragmented, contradictory, frustrating, and most of all, ineffective. But we get on with it, even though it may be unclear what philosophy or principle drives our activities. We fail to ask ourselves:

- Who are these people whom we move, feed, and medicate?
- Where are their families?
- What are we doing for them?
- Why am I so tired and frustrated?
- What is the plan?
- Is there a plan?

A great many competent people are employed in providing health care to elderly people. New and renovated institutions are developed every day. Policies and procedures, standards and regulations, and guidelines are being written by the ton. Health policies are being developed. Budgets are being formulated; committees, associations, societies, teams, and consultants are being formed, all of them constantly meeting and conferencing. In short, there is a fierce focus on dementing diseases and what we should do about them.

But the bottom line in all of this activity is very simple. It is not a policy bottom line, financial bottom line, industrial relations bottom line, or regulatory bottom line. The definitive bottom line is:

- How well are they doing—the elderly people entrusted to our care?
- What is the quality of their daily existence?
- How are their families managing?

These questions must echo in our institutions, our policies, and our minds as we go about our daily responsibilities, no matter what level of work we do with people who suffer from dementia. Furthermore, the question, "How do my personal actions affect the lives of the people whose care is entrusted to me?" needs to be asked by researchers, ministers of health, housekeepers who shine the floors in care facilities, board members of societies that support and educate families, visiting homemakers, members of curriculum committees at universities, family caregivers, congregations in churches, dieticians, neighbors, union shop stewards, directors of care, grandchildren, and health care staff of institutions.

Until a medical cure for progressive dementing illnesses like Alzheimer's disease is found, the most effective way to help people who suffer the effects of such illnesses is to develop appropriate care systems. If the way we care for people with dementia is not a way that we ourselves could tolerate—if they are not comfortable; if they are anxious, confused, frightened, frustrated, or restrained; if they are abused, crushed, or empty—then we must change the way we are doing things, for the sake of afflicted people, for their families, for care providers, for our communities. To do this we need a map or model.

Developing a Health Care Paradigm

A model for the practice of health care develops from several elements:
- a *philosophy* based on the values and beliefs we hold sacred, personally, professionally, and as members of society; and
- a *body of knowledge,* compounded of data, observations, and analysis.

Our philosophy and knowledge base enable us to develop:
- a *frame of reference,* which is the assumptions and concepts that shape the way we work; and
- a *conceptual model* that helps us understand why we carry out a given type of practice.

On the basis of our conceptual model, we propose:
- our *model of practice* or how we do what we do, such as the strategies and activities that translate our conceptual model into reality; and
- the *expected results* or objectives of our model of practice. Outcomes are promises about what our model of practice will accomplish.

In life each man paints his own portrait. And there is nothing but the portrait. It is not what you would have done, could have done, or should have done. . . . [It is] just what you did.

—JEAN PAUL SARTRE

A model or paradigm of care, therefore, is the map we use to help us design and deliver a certain kind of health care. Many different models of care have been used or proposed. Several are currently in use, each based on a different set of principles or theories about care and treatment:

- The *custodial care model* focuses on maintaining the physical condition of a person in care for as long as possible.
- The *biomedical acute care model* centers on the treatment and elimination of symptoms which are signs of pathology. The emphasis is on efficiency and speedy resolution of the problem. Staff is trained to be emotionally neutral and objective. The primary interventions are invasive strategies, drugs, and surgery. Body and mind are regarded as separate entities, although this view is beginning to change. The acute care environment is institutional and technologically intensive. The sick person is regarded as a "patient" who is dependent upon professional staff for information and problem resolution. In acute care situations, the labor force is divided along professional or territorial lines, which is very costly. This model of care has been very successful in the treatment of physical illness. The biomedical model is very costly.
- The *functional independence model* is concerned with a person's ability to function socially and psychologically with physical well-being.
- The *therapeutic model*'s goal is a person's successful integration of physical and social achievement.
- The *prosthetic model of care,* which I developed, is based on the premise that appropriate care can be given only when there has been an accurate definition of the deficit a person is experiencing. Only then can the macro-environment (people, programs, and physical space) be organized into a *prosthesis of care* designed to compensate for the person's deficits, to support existing or residual function, and to maximize quality of life.

In this chapter we have been talking about various models of practice now in use, and the need to change them to respond to changing

GENTLECARE
PROSTHETIC MODEL OF CARE FOR DEMENTIA

Philosophy
- Elderly people have value.
- People with dementia suffer from a complex disease.
- Independence is better than dependence.
- Internal control is better than external control.
- Individuals have a right to a meaningful existence, whatever their level of development or health problem.
- People with dementia have diminished resources to control or direct their behavior.
- Care providers can change their behavior to be more effective.

Knowledge
- Precise diagnosis and identification of the dementing illness and its effects.
- Social history and context of people with dementia is known.

Gentlecare Frame of Reference
- Behavior can be affected by external stimulus.
- Behavior occurs within a context.

Conceptual Model
- Performance deficits can be compensated for by a prosthesis of support composed of people, programs, and physical space.

Model of Practice
- Know the person and the disease.
- Engage the family in therapeutic partnership.
- Educate the therapeutic agent(s).
- Identify and control external influences, and modify strategies.
- Modify the environment.
- Design meaningful opportunities for activity.
- Evaluate.

Outcomes
- Behavioral change can be achieved.
- Behavior can be shaped, changed, generalized, and/or extinguished.
- Functional levels can be altered to enhance independence.
- Personal resources can be preserved.
- Costs can be reduced.

FIGURE 2-1

clinical issues and profiles. If we are to accomplish such change, we will have to ask ourselves:

- How does transformation from one paradigm to another happen?
- What can be usefully retained of the old models, and what must be created anew?

T.S. Kuhn, in his groundbreaking book, *The Structure of Scientific Revolutions* (University of Chicago Press, 1974), notes:

> Since new paradigms are born from old ones, they ordinarily incorporate much of the vocabulary and apparatus, both conceptual and manipulative, that the traditional paradigm had previously employed. But they seldom employ these borrowed elements in quite the traditional way. Within the new paradigm, old terms, concepts and experiments fall into what we must call, though the term is not quite right, a misunderstanding between the two competing schools.

The Gentlecare Prosthetic Life Care System is an example of a prosthetic model of care. It provides a new map that can lead us through the maze-like process of dementia care.

> *A human being is part of the whole, called by us the "Universe," a part limited in time and space. He experiences himself, his thoughts and feelings, as something separated from the rest—a kind of optical delusion of his consciousness. This delusion is a kind of prison for us, restricting us to our personal desires and to affection for a few persons nearest to us. Our task must be to free ourselves from this prison by widening our circles of compassion to embrace all living creatures and the whole of nature in its beauty.*
>
> —ALBERT EINSTEIN

CHARACTERISTICS OF THE
PROSTHETIC HEALTH CARE PARADIGM

- The prosthetic model of care focuses on patterns of behavior and causes of problems.
- Human values, conversation, and connections are emphasized by staff whose method of caring is the major component of therapy.
- Noninvasive tools and techniques are used, with significant reliance on an appropriate person/environment fit; the focus is on the use of human interaction (music, massage, hugs, pets, walks, talks).
- Integration of body, mind, and spirit is critical to the care approach.
- Environments are simple, normalized, therapeutic, and prosthetic.
- Since many of the symptoms of dementing illness cannot be treated, the emphasis is on identifying and supporting remaining function.
- The objective of dementia care is to assist and support the client and his family.
- The social context is vital; professionals, families, and communities work in therapeutic partnership.
- All staff are the principal therapeutic agents; their way of caring is the major component of therapy.
- There is a mix of jobs by small groups.

FIGURE 2-2

3

An Overview of Gentlecare

My wish, indeed my continuing passion, would be not to point the
finger in judgement, but to part a curtain, that invisible shadow
that falls between people; the veil of indifference to each other's
presence, each other's wonder, each other's human plight.
—Eudora Welty,
American Author

Gentlecare is a prosthetic system of dementia care designed to change
the experience of a dementing illness such as Alzheimer's disease for
those afflicted person, their families, and professional caregivers. The
system is based on my personal experience, as well as on the experience of hundreds of family and professional caregivers who, like me,
are searching for more appropriate solutions to the devastating problems raised by dementia.

The challenge of providing appropriate services to older people with
dementing illnesses preoccupies health care planners and practitioners alike. As knowledge of those illnesses grows, it is becoming clear
that current health systems, policies, and models of care not only compromise quality of life for people with dementia; they are sources of *ia-*
trogenic illness as well. Iatrogenic illness is illness caused by the care,
the environment, or factors other than the disease. It results in accelerated loss of function for people suffering from dementia, and therefore
in excessive dependency on other people; ultimately such illness esca-
lates the costs of care.

In addition, current health care practices distance family caregivers
from their loved ones, causing untold anguish and frustration. Profes-

sional health care providers also report ever-increasing levels of personal stress, physical injury, and job dissatisfaction.

Gentlecare offers a positive approach not only to the relentless progress of dementing illness, but also to the unnecessary dysfunction and heartache of iatrogenic illness. The system is rooted in a recognition of the person with dementia as a unique and special human being with a rich history and a difficult future. This person is acknowledged to be experiencing devastating problems, and so deserves appropriate and compassionate assistance with the life challenges to come.

Unfortunately, there is a malignant myth in dementia care that family caregivers may take responsibility for people with dementia for the first few years of the illness, but then professional caregivers need to take over. On occasion, families have been encouraged to disappear from the caregiving scene, or to "have a rest." When this happens, family members sometimes feel impotent or unnecessary and may sever their relationship with the afflicted family member. This causes untold anguish and frustration.

In the Gentlecare system the person suffering from dementia is thought of as part of a family, and any intervention takes this into account. Gentlecare emphasizes that whole families, not just individuals, suffer from Alzheimer's disease. Effective dementia care must acknowledge the power of family by supporting and assisting family members, and involving them in the care process. If there is no existing family, it is sometimes necessary to create an artificial or surrogate family.

The Concept of a Prosthesis of Care: People, Programs, and Physical Space

Gentlecare is a comprehensive program designed to prepare professional staff and family caregivers to care for persons with primary progressive dementias. The system is applicable in acute care institutions, long-term care facilities, and day care programs; and it changes the way family caregivers see their role in a demented person's own home.

Gentlecare advocates a major shift in focus away from a concentration on the behaviors of the person with dementia, and toward an adjustment of the physical and social environment in which the person must operate. It involves a significant paradigm shift in the way we think and act in caring for people with dementia.

This process begins by ensuring that staff and family members clearly understand the clinical process and implications of progressive dementia. The emphasis is on an awareness of the afflicted person's relationships and life context, in which the person lives, rather than on crisis intervention. Family members and staff are helped to identify and remove stressors in the environment of the person with dementia. They are encouraged to develop effective strategies and programs that will help the individual live more comfortably within the environment.

Gentlecare assists staff and families to evaluate the functional strengths and deficits of the person, and provides them with assessment methods, criteria for admission to special care units, strategies for problem-solving and stress reduction, and tools to alleviate troubling behaviors.

One of the most prevalent medical problems of our times is iatrogenic illness. It results from surgical complications, wrong medication, side effects of drugs or other treatments, and the debilitating effects of hospitalizaion.

—THE AQUARIAN CONSPIRACY

Caregivers learn how to maximize the afflicted person's existing abilities by designing and developing exciting activities and helpful programs, and integrating supportive care patterns into daily life. Suggestions are made for communication techniques that family caregivers and professionals can use with people experiencing dementia.

The Gentlecare system advocates a therapeutic partnership among care facilities, families, and community volunteers. Suggestions are offered on how to involve families and community volunteers in assisting with dementia care, creating a modified community for the afflicted person within the health care system.

Touch is the most powerful positive intervention.

Gentlecare advocates adapted "work" therapy strategies to help improve the demented person's quality of life. Such strategies can provide

Delta Habilitation Centre, Delta, BC, Canada.
This building was designed specifically to provide dedicated indoor and outdoor living space for people with dementia. It is composed of four living spaces, each of which opens onto a therapeutic garden.

people with meaningful activity while showing respect for former lifestyles and roles. The Gentlecare system accommodates and supports existing levels of function and development, rather than requiring people with dementia to perform in ways that are no longer possible.

Gentlecare is a system that focuses on using the *macro-environment* to achieve effective dementia care. Methods are outlined for developing prosthetic physical environments—both indoors and outdoors—that support rather than challenge dysfunctional persons. Suggestions are made for modifying existing environments, as well as for designing and developing purpose-built facilities. Gentlecare designs a prosthesis of care or *enviro-match* between people with dementing illness and:
- the physical space in which they live;
- their daily activities; and
- the significant people with whom they interact.

People with dementia are not asked to perform activities in ways they no longer can. Contrast this with the usual care facility environment. Most care facilities provide communal living arrangements, set up within buildings that are institutional in design and frequently technologically focused. Inside those buildings, an unbelievable array of ac-

Although I have sickness in me, if the focus is on my wellness, allow it to overshadow my sickness.

—AUTHOR UNKNOWN

CHAPTER
THREE

tivities takes place—maintenance and housekeeping, education, life-saving health care, public functions—all happening alongside the daily activities of people dealing with dementia. It is hard for us to even imagine our own lives being played out in the midst of such a hive of bewildering activity.

PROSTHESIS

A device or artificial structure (either external or implanted) that substitutes for, or supplements, a missing or defective part.

In the Gentlecare system, the environment is regarded as more than just the physical space in which people live. The macro-environment of people with progressive dementing illness consists of people, programs, and physical space, working in a dynamic interaction. The macro-environment forms the total context in which the person with dementing illness must live and function throughout the course of the disease.

Gentlecare introduces the concept of the *prosthesis of care,* in which the three components—people, programs, and physical space—work in harmony to produce a support, or *prosthesis* for the person with de-mentia. Such a prosthesis compensates for the deficits created by a de-menting illness.

The replacement of physical body parts by prosthetic devices is a well-accepted procedure in health care. If someone sustains a spinal cord injury, for example, a wheelchair is prescribed to compensate for the resulting paralysis. With this prosthesis, the injured person can re-gain control over life; without the prosthesis, the person is dependent on others and quite helpless.

Dementia destroys people's ability to manage their needs and be in control in a way that closely parallels the effects of physical paralysis, since it, too, makes them dependent on others for daily care. Just as a wheelchair can recreate mobility for a spinal injury patient, an appro-priate prosthesis can give a person with dementia an improved quality of life. Gentlecare manipulates those three vital components—people, programs, and physical space—in ways that assist and support people through the course of a dementing illness.

People: The First Element of the Prosthesis of Care

Of the three components of the person's macro-environment, by far the most critical is people. The person with dementia is surrounded by people, including the key family caregiver (usually a spouse or a mid-life daughter or son) and other significant family members. They form a vital support system that must be maintained throughout the disease process—regardless of where the person with dementia lives. Professional care providers form an artificial support system that needs to be specifically focused. And people with dementia are forced to live with large numbers of other ill people, which can make life very challenging. In addition to these key individuals, at any point in time the dysfunctional person's "home" may be invaded by any number of other people, such as volunteers, visitors, or administrative staff.

All these people can either be agents of help or forces of destruction in their impact on the health of a person with dementia. Their beliefs, attitudes, and language shape the life of the person with dementia; their level of education, skills, and judgement can make all the difference in the world. In Gentlecare, people are the essential therapeutic agents of dementia care.

Programs: The Second Element of the Prosthesis of Care

Programs include everything the person with dementia does or has done to him, in a 24-hour cycle. In place of the standard rigid activity schedule driven by artificial wake-up times, sleep times, and meal times, interspersed with sporadic social or recreational activities, Gentlecare uses *all* activity in the life of the person with dementia to enhance his experience and ensure he leads a meaningful life.

Programs designed for persons with dementia are most effective when they are an integral part of daily life, rather than "add-ons" or "take-outs," or activities parachuted into the daily routine. Programming that focuses on and supports self-care, communication, intimacy, relaxation, stress reduction, competency, and former life roles often has magical effects on persons with dementia. All program initiatives should be designed to support and celebrate the existing strengths of people in care.

Physical Space: The Third Element of the Prosthesis of Care

The physical environment of people with dementia needs to be simple, normalized, and therapeutic. It must be space designed to be lived in, and must resonate with familiar personal memorabilia.

Experience has shown that areas dedicated for the use of people with dementia most effectively support their needs. Many design features can help to enhance function and quality of life, such as secure perimeters; indoor and outdoor walking paths; appropriate wayfinding cues and signage; multiple small social and dining areas; avoidance of distracting patterns; reduction of glare, noise, and confusion; and family cluster living arrangements.

It has been said that the challenge for people with dementia is not in facing death—it is facing life.

The Impact of the Prosthesis of Care

The task of helping people with the formidable cognitive damage caused by dementing illness is daunting. Gentlecare takes on this task by first identifying the disease, and then assessing the specific deficits in function caused by the disease at a given moment in time. Then Gentlecare designs a personal prosthesis of care for each person with dementia, to help each of them manage daily life challenges. The components of the prosthesis of care—people, programs, and physical space—are not costly add-ons to existing programs; they are part of existing basic health care services. However, Gentlecare organizes those components differently, so that they support—rather than challenge—the person with cognitive impairment.

In Gentlecare, people, programs, and physical space are set up in creative, dynamic interaction. Gentlecare prostheses have as many variations as there are people needing help or people offering help. For example:

- In a Gentlecare unit, maintenance workers don't just walk into a room to fix a tap or hang a picture. As members of the Gentlecare team, they are aware of working in a person's "home." Therefore, they engage in conversation with the person with dementia, identify the project, ask for the host's opinion—in other words, attempt to involve the host, however marginally. Thanks is given for any contribution to the work, thereby enhancing self-esteem.

- In hospitals and health care facilities, public address systems are used to call people to telephones, make announcements, and alert people to emergencies. This practice is not viewed favorably in Gentlecare units, since sudden, loud voices issuing from the PA system are frightening, disorienting, intrusive, and confusing for people struggling with cognitive impairment. A Gentlecare environment eliminates this stress factor, and uses personal pagers or written messages instead of public address systems.

It works! It works!

—A CARE AIDE

- It is common practice in health care institutions for the night shift staff to get people up and dressed before the day shift staff arrives, in order to "get a head start on the day's work." This is one of the most unsettling of all institutional practices. Gentlecare units, in contrast, adapt the morning wake-up routine so that older, cognitively impaired people can wake-up naturally. They are not rushed, they are helped to enjoy the beginning of their day, and they are appropriately oriented and prepared for the coming day's activities.

This is really common sense!

—A DIRECTOR OF
NURSING CARE

These are but three examples of different ways to help. Gentlecare is a simple, common sense, affordable, "do-able" approach to care that can be practiced by family caregivers, professional caregivers, support staff, volunteers, friends, and neighbors alike.

The Gentlecare system enables people who are ill to lead tolerable, even comfortable, lives, avoiding confrontation and crises despite the devastation of their disease. It gives life back to family caregivers, and protects them against threats to their own health by helping them avoid crises.

Gentlecare empowers professional care providers, offering them new ways to address problems in their workplace. It reduces accidents and injuries, improves staff morale, and puts joy back into the workplace.

The Theater of Gentlecare

People often ask me how I think of solutions to the endless number of problems that arise in caring for people with dementia—how I visualize Gentlecare in action within a care facility. I often think of Gentlecare as a theatrical performance, one in which staff members, family caregivers, volunteers, and the people with dementia are engaged in the presentation of an ongoing play.

I see the people with dementia as the actors in the play. I see the unit manager, the care coordinator, or supervisor as the director of the play—the person who pulls all the bits and pieces together to keep momentum. I see the people who work in activities and recreation, the custodial staff and volunteers, as the stage crew who prepare the stage and sets in which the play takes place.

The care aides and others who give direct care act as prompters. I imagine that each person with dementia has a prompter—a care aide, a family caregiver, a volunteer, or one of the support staff. The prompter is there to keep the actors (people with dementia) on track by giving cues, reminding them of lines, and giving them the information they need to carry out their daily "performance." The play takes place throughout all the working hours.

Everyone has to know the care plan, which is the manuscript for the play. The "director/unit manager" has the master copy of the script/care plan, and everyone has the same script, and everyone follows it. The lines and the stage directions are all there.

If a change to the script is proposed by the director, one of the stage crew, or a prompter, or if a script change is made because of a change in the condition of the actor, it is the director's responsibility to ensure that the suggested change is suitable and effective. The director must also ensure that the whole crew knows what the change is, and that it is written into the script.

OUTCOMES OF GENTLECARE

Institutions and families using the Gentlecare Prosthetic Life Care System report the following outcomes:
- improved levels of functioning in the person with dementia
- greater participation in self-care activities
- increased spontaneous socialization and communication
- reduced non-cognitive and assaultive behaviors
- less wandering
- fewer arguments and altercations
- fewer episodes of catastrophic behavior
- reduced incontinence
- improved family comfort and participation in care
- accelerated volunteer and community involvement
- trends indicating cost savings

FIGURE 3-1

At any given point in the day, one or more actors are on stage performing an activity. They could be having a bath, eating a meal, going to an exercise program, or waking up and getting dressed for the day. The people with dementia are helped to perform that activity.

When that scene is completed, they go off stage and rest, in the same way that actors perform a scene and then exit and rest before they come back on stage. The job of the director is to facilitate the whole theatrical event and to make sure that every person with dementia has a prompter; that each actor has the necessary information and support to perform appropriately; and that the whole environment supports the role that each one plays.

Every single person on the unit—physician, board member, housekeeping staff, visitor, nurse, care aide, or rehabilitation staff member—has to be aware of what play is being presented each day. They must know the actors' abilities and their roles. They must know what kind of props and sets are needed to perform properly. It's up to them to prepare all that—to support, encourage, and inspire people with dementia to give the best performances of which they are capable.

I feel as if a light bulb had gone on in my head. Now, when I look at the person with dementia through different eyes, I know how to help him.

—A PHYSICIAN

4

Why Do They Do What They Do?

I'm not stupid!
I have Alzheimer's disease!
        —a person with Alzheimer's

Fundamental to the design of the Gentlecare program or any dementia care program is an understanding of dementing disease. Dementia is the loss of intellectual functions—such as thinking, remembering, and reasoning—of sufficient severity to interfere with a person's daily functioning.

Dementia is not a disease in itself, but rather a group of symptoms that may accompany certain diseases or physical conditions. The degree of damage and rate of progression of dementias varies, depending on both the cause of the symptoms and the particular individual affected. Some of the more familiar diseases that produce dementia include Alzheimer's disease, multi-infarct dementia, Huntington's disease, and sometimes Parkinson's disease.

Dementia can present in either acute or chronic forms. Acute dementias (or acute deliriums) are metabolic or systemic in nature. They respond to treatment and the damage can often be reversed. Chronic dementias, on the other hand, for the most part cannot be treated successfully, since the damage that creates the dementia is structural and irreversible. There is permanent damage to brain tissue.

Alzheimer's disease (pronounced *Allts' hi-merz*) was first described by Dr. Alois Alzheimer in 1907. It is the most common of the dementing disorders, and is a progressive, degenerative disease that attacks brain cells and results in impaired memory, thinking, and behavior. The rate of progression, as with all dementias, varies from one person to another.

> **ALZHEIMER'S DISEASE**
>
> The time from diagnosis to death, on average, is 8 years, but may range from 5 to 20 years.
>
> Ten to fifteen percent of persons with Alzheimer's disease hallucinate or have delusions.
>
> One in ten people with Alzheimer's disease has seizures.
>
> —*US News and World Report*, August 1991

Not infrequently, when we first meet people with dementia, we know very little about the essential person behind the disease. It is not possible to treat such people appropriately until we know the answers to these basic questions:

- Who is this man or woman?
- What is important to him or her?
- Does he have different perceptions than I?
- How does she feel?

More often than not, professional caregivers know very little about the actual process of dementing disease, or how far the disease has progressed in an individual. Families rarely have the information they need to be able to react appropriately to their loved one's actions. Caregivers, both lay and professional, need to be aware that there is a direct correlation between the nature of disease the person is experiencing and the behavior they are exhibiting.

Behavior—especially problem behavior—does not occur at random or in isolation. Behavior follows a course that corresponds to the disease process. People suffering from a dementing disease behave the way they do because the disease has evolved to a particular stage. The symptoms and unusual behaviors that result from brain damage

DEMENTIA

Types

Acute/Delirium	Chronic
• responds to treatment	• cannot be reversed
• is metabolic/systemic	• structural damage
• damage may be reversed	• irreversible damage to the brain tissue

Causes

• drug toxicity	• Alzheimer's disease
• alcoholism	• multi-infarct/vascular
• dehydration	• Huntington's disease
• hypothyroidism	• Pick's disease
• vitamin B12 deficit	• Parkinson's disease
• depression	• Korsakoff's syndrome
• sensory deficits	• AIDS-related dementia
• infections	
• congestive heart failure	
• malnutrition	
• stress	
• compounded loss	

(Diseases may occur in any combination.)

FIGURE 4-1

correspond to the particular function of the damaged area of the brain. In fact, these effects are sometimes referred to as "physiological maps" of the brain, since they indicate what area of the brain has been affected.

The behavior of people with dementia is exacerbated by stressors such as terror, confusion, frustration, misconceptions, disorientation, and (justifiable) anger. Their actions are seldom premeditated, but are based on feelings rather than thought. *Their behavior is the best behavior they are capable of, given the circumstances they find themselves in.* Behavior is the window to a person's mind, and must be studied very carefully.

Most caregiver action or care plans developed for people with dementia are behavior driven: that is, a care strategy, intervention, or procedure is initiated in response to the fact that a person with dementia has behaved in a certain way—rather than as a response to the functional implications of the disease that caused the behavior.

For example, consider a person who is observed to be walking randomly. A typical behavior-driven strategy is to get the person to sit down and be quiet. But suppose the wandering person is trying to find a drink? As Alzheimer's disease progresses, the part of the brain that regulates body thirst is damaged, and people with Alzheimer's disease frequently experience terrible thirst. Suppose the person is trying to find a drink while disoriented and confused by a complex environment?

If our care strategy has been to ask the person to sit down or we have ensured compliance through the use of restraints, how effective have we been in meeting that person's actual needs? Thirst is a powerful need, and the person may be quite persistent in trying to quench it. How much will the control strategies need to be escalated to ensure that the person stays put? Will that require a verbal request, physical restraint, or control by drugs?

Alzheimer's disease progresses without visible "markers". We must therefore rely on the behaviors we can observe to give clues about a person's functional abilities. Only with that information can we build a plan of care that addresses the person's needs appropriately. If in devising a care plan strategy we fail to make the vital connection between the person, the disease he is experiencing, and the behaviors he is exhibiting as a result, then we will likely fall far short of giving appropriate care to that person. Making that connection changes the way we deliver dementia care.

Behavior is the window to a person's mind. It allows us to understand why a person acts the way they do.

Planning Care Using the Gentlecare Formula

The Gentlecare formula is a method of organizing thinking and action based on a comprehensive evaluation of the needs of a person with dementia—rather than on a reactive response to the person's behavior.

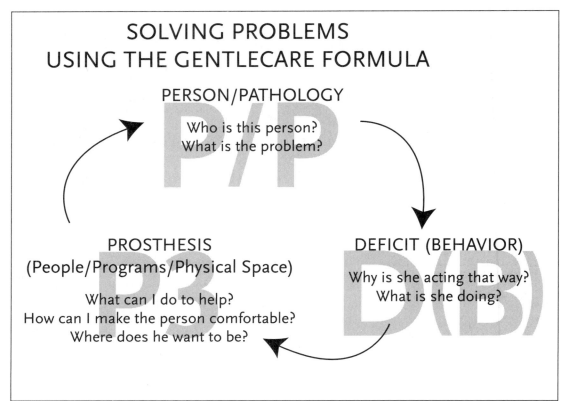

SOLVING PROBLEMS
USING THE GENTLECARE FORMULA

PERSON/PATHOLOGY

Who is this person?
What is the problem?

DEFICIT (BEHAVIOR)

Why is she acting that way?
What is she doing?

PROSTHESIS
(People/Programs/Physical Space)

What can I do to help?
How can I make the person comfortable?
Where does he want to be?

FIGURE 4-2

The formula helps us to remember that all intervention should be designed for the individual, and based on the specific pathology the person is experiencing (person/pathology). Next, the deficit in functioning caused by the disease is reviewed; this is done by observing and monitoring the deficit the individual is experiencing as manifested or exhibited by his behavior (D(B)). Once the problem has been correctly identified, a prosthesis of care strategy can be developed (prosthesis). In Gentlecare this prosthesis consists of supportive people, meaningful strategies, and a residential environment that supports the person.

It should be noted that the Gentlecare formula works from any point in the triangle (see Figure 4-2). For example, we can observe a behavior and ask what deficit that represents before we plan strategies. It is not uncommon in health care facilities to observe elderly people engaging in unusual sexual behavior. When staff encounter such behavior, it is helpful if they are aware that such activity on the part of elderly people is usually due to damage to the part of the brain that provides emotional and sexual control, rather than being malevolent premeditated behavior. This information helps to devise an appropriate response rather than a judgemental or punitive one.

Alternatively, we can use the formula to examine the appropriateness of the prosthesis given the particular deficit of the individual in care. For example, if the strategy in a health care facility is to wake, groom, and dress individuals early in the morning, we might ask: Given an individual's personal preferences and habits, together with the damage caused by the disease, is this stressful care strategy contributing to this person's behavior? Could we devise a better strategy?

Understanding "Childlike" Behaviors

As discussed in Chapter 1, Dr. Barry Reisberg suggests that people suffering from a dementing disease experience loss of skills in a sequence not unlike that which a child follows in the development of skills, but in reverse order. As a result, although people with dementia are *not* children, they are childlike. We must respect them as elders at all times; however, if we want to help them appropriately, we need to understand that they are losing the abilities we normally assume older people have. Consequently, their behavior as adults may appear to be inappropriate or irresponsible.

Behind the idea
And the reality
Between the motion
And the Act
Falls the shadow
—T.S. ELIOT,
THE HOLLOW MEN

> I REMEMBER AN *elderly lady saying to me, "Moyra, caring for my husband is like running around after an eight-year-old all day! I'm exhausted." And of course, given the stage of illness, his behavior did resemble that of an eight-year-old child.*

The following scale clearly outlines the performance deficits that a person with dementia will experience. It is very helpful as a guide to care planning.

REVERSE ORDER OF DEVELOPMENT SCALE

APPROX. AGE	ABILITIES	STAGE OF DISEASE
12 Yrs	Hold a job	Borderline
8–12 Yrs	Handle simple finances	Early (Stage 2)
5–7 Yrs	Select proper clothing	Moderate (Stage 3 & 4)
5 Yrs	Put on clothes Personal grooming	Severe (Stage 5)
4 Yrs	Go to toilet unaided	
3–4½ Yrs	Control urine	
3 Yrs	Control bowels	
15 Months	Speak 5–6 words	Late (Stage 6)
1 Yr	Speak 1 word	
1 Yr	Walk	
6–9 Months	Sit up	
2–3 Months	Smile	

ABILITIES INCREASE WITH AGE

ABILITIES DECREASE WITH DISEASE

FIGURE 4-3

Reference: Dr. Barry Reisberg

The information provided in the Global Deterioration Scale, page 39-41, helps families and other care providers to understand the stages of Alzheimer's disease.

THE GLOBAL DETERIORATION SCALE FOR ASSESSMENT OF PRIMARY DEGENERATIVE DEMENTIA

Level	Clinical Characteristics
I No cognitive decline	No subjective complaint of memory deficit. No memory deficit evident on clinical interview.
II Very mild cognitive decline (forgetfulness)	Subjective complaints of memory deficit, most frequently in the following areas: (a) forgetting where one has placed familiar objects; (b) forgetting names one formerly knew well. No objective evidence of memory deficit on clinical interview. No objective deficit in employment or social situations. Appropriate concern with respect to symptomatology.
III Mild cognitive decline (early confusional)	Early clear-cut deficits. Manifestations in more than one of the following areas: (a) patient may have gotten lost while traveling to an unfamiliar destination; (b) co-workers become aware of patient's relatively poor performance; (c) word- and name-finding deficit becomes evident to intimates; (d) patient may read a passage or book and retain little material; (e) patient may demonstrate decreased facility in remembering names upon introduction to new people; (f) patient may have lost or misplaced an object of value; (g) concentration deficit may be evident in clinical testing. Objective evidence of memory deficit obtained only with intensive interview. Decreased performance in demanding employment and social settings. Denial begins to become manifest in patient. Mild to moderate anxiety accompanies symptoms.

FIGURE 4-4

IV Moderate cognitive decline (late confusional)	Clear-cut deficits on careful clinical interview. Deficit manifest in the following areas: (a) decreased knowledge of current and recent events; (b) may exhibit some deficit in memory of personal history; (c) concentration deficit elicited on serial subtractions; (d) decreased ability to travel to familiar locations. Inability to perform complex tasks. Denial is a dominant defense mechanism. Flattening of affect and withdrawal from challenging situations occurs.
V Moderate-severe cognitive decline (early dementia)	Patient can no longer survive without assistance. During interview, patient unable to recall major, relevant aspects of his current life—e.g., address or telephone number of many years' standing, the names of close family members (such as grandchildren) or the name of the high school or college from which they graduated. Frequently some disorientation to time (date, day of the week, season, etc.) or to place. An educated person may have difficulty counting backward from 40 by 4's or from 20 by 2's. Persons at this stage retain knowledge of many major facts about themselves and others. They invariably know their own names and generally know the names of their spouses and children. They require no assistance with toileting or eating, but may have difficulty choosing proper clothing to wear.
VI Severe cognitive decline (middle dementia)	Many patients at this stage occasionally forget the name of the spouse on whom they are entirely dependent for survival. Will be largely unaware of all recent events and experiences in their lives. Retain some knowledge of their past lives, but this is very sketchy. Generally unaware of their surroundings, the year, the season, etc. May have difficulty counting from 10 both backward and (sometimes) for-

	ward. Will require some assistance with activities of daily living (e.g., may become incontinent). Will require assistance with travel but occasionally will display ability to find familiar locations. Diurnal rhythm frequently disturbed. Almost always recall their own names. Frequently continue to be able to distinguish from unfamiliar people in their environment. Personality and emotional changes occur; these are quite variable, and include (a) delusional behaviour (e.g., patient may accuse spouse of being an imposter, may talk to imaginary figures, or to their own reflections in the mirror); (b) obsessive symptoms appear—the demented person may continually repeat simple cleaning activities; (c) anxiety symptoms, agitation, and even previously non-existent violent behavior may occur; (d) cognitive abulia occurs (loss of willpower because an individual cannot carry a thought long enough to determine a purposeful course of action).
VII Very severe cognitive decline (late dementia)	All verbal abilities are lost. Frequently there is no speech at all, only grunting. Incontinent of urine, requires assistance with toileting and feeding. Loses basic psychomotor skills (e.g., the ability to walk). It appears the brain is no longer able to tell the body what to do. Generalized and cortical neurological signs and symptoms are frequently present.

Reisberg, B., Ferris, S.H., Leon, M.J. and Cook, T., "The Global Deterioration Scale for the Assessment of Primary Degenerative Dementia," *American Journal of Psychiatry,* 1992 139: 1136–1139

PARTS OF THE BRAIN
AFFECTED BY ALZHEIMER'S

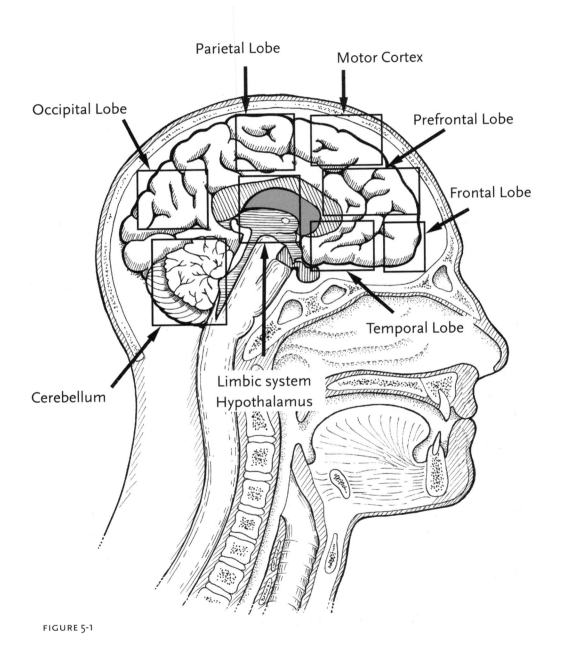

Parietal Lobe

Motor Cortex

Occipital Lobe

Prefrontal Lobe

Frontal Lobe

Temporal Lobe

Cerebellum

Limbic system
Hypothalamus

FIGURE 5-1

5

The Clinical Course of Alzheimer's Disease

I think, therefore I am.
—Rene Descartes

The Gentlecare system emphasizes the need for family members and professional caregivers to understand the nature of the diseases experienced by the people in their care. Each dementing disease has its own progression, which produces its own sequence of behaviors. I'll use Alzheimer's disease to illustrate the course of dementia, because it is the dementing disease seen most often. It affects every area of the brain, and so illustrates all the problems associated with any of the dementias, such as vascular illness, Parkinson's disease, chronic alcoholism, and others. Understanding the pathology of Alzheimer's disease helps caregivers and family members to understand behaviors caused by any of the dementing illnesses.

What follows in this chapter is an explanation of the effects that Alzheimer's disease has on brain tissue, and consequently on brain function and behavior.

First Signs: Damage to the Limbic System

In Alzheimer's disease, the first nerve cells to die are those in the area deep within the brain known as the *limbic system*. The limbic system is responsible for memory and emotional control. Memory processing

LIMBIC SYSTEM
Damage

FIGURE 5-2

may take place throughout the whole brain, but certain areas within and bordering the limbic system, particularly the hippocampus, appear to be vital to memory. Control of sexuality is also thought to be located there.

As this area of the brain becomes filled with the characteristic tangles and plaques of Alzheimer's disease, memories of the recent past fade and the memory processing function becomes compromised. Over time, more long-standing memories will fade.

As the limbic system dies, affected people give evidence of emotional instability. They experience rapid changes of mood, alternating between a flat affect and euphoria. They are unable to control their anxiety, and switch rapidly from states of fearfulness to restlessness to irritability to aggressiveness—eventually lapsing into helplessness. At this point in the disease process, the following behaviors arise:

- People will act tearful and anxious.
- They may act depressed and suspicious.
- They are certainly terrified and frustrated.
- They may have verbal outbursts.
- They are agitated.
- They engage in seemingly purposeless activity, wandering to and fro, trying to make sense of what is happening to them.
- They are unable to retain the meaning of written words after reading.
- They misplace objects and then become suspicious that others may be taking things from them, or hiding them.
- They may be sexually active.

To build a prosthesis for people with these problems, caregivers need to be understanding, supportive, and provide information as often as necessary—as often as the afflicted person requests it. The person with dementia needs therapy for depression and/or anxiety. All stresses on the patient, and demands or expectations placed on them, must be modified. Life activities need to be simplified. The family needs education and assistance in terms of sexual issues.

Damage Spreads to the Parietal Area

Damage eventually spreads upward to the parietal area of the cortex. The *parietal lobe* is the center for spatial perception, sensory integration, and concentration. As this area of the brain becomes affected, people with Alzheimer's lose the ability to recognize places, objects, and people (faces). At this stage—

- They easily become disoriented and lost.
- They begin to lose the ability to recognize familiar sensory stimuli, a condition called *agnosia*.
- They have problems identifying objects in terms of their function.
- They begin to have problems identifying people—especially those of a different generation, or people they do not see often (called *visual agnosia*). Families need to understand why the person may not recognize them.
- They may experience imaginary visual images (hallucinations).
- One in ten people with dementia will have grand mal or petit mal seizures.
- They lose the ability to concentrate or focus. This means a person with Alzheimer's disease will have trouble maintaining attention and will be very easily distracted. Noises or activity in the environment can therefore interfere with the person's ability to listen, process information, and perform a given activity. At this point in the disease, stress of any kind is toxic. This is a critical deficit.
- As spatial perception declines, they begin to lose the ability to locate certain parts of the body. Activities like grooming, or following directions in exercise groups, become difficult.
- Deteriorating hand skills often makes it difficult for them to carry out activities of daily living, such as crafts, cooking, and so on. This is the beginning of what is called *constructional apraxia*.
- They begin to experience deterioration in speech organization. The person with dementia has difficulty interpreting symbols, and thus cannot benefit from signs or notes. As a result, driving (for example) becomes dangerous.
- They have difficulty with syntax (the rules governing the arrange-

PARIETAL LOBE
Damage

FIGURE 5-3

ment of words in sentences). These problems are referred to as *auditory agnosia.*

- They have problems in touch interpretation *(tactile agnosia);* they can't identify an object unless they can see it. Care needs to be taken with sharp objects.

To build a prosthesis for people with these problems, caregivers must assist the person by "grounding" them and helping them to focus and concentrate. This is accomplished by reducing stress, noise, glare, confusion, and rush in the living environment. The person's tasks and environment are simplified. Good wayfinding cues are needed, such as written cues, pictures, and familiar objects. All the person's senses need to be involved for orientation. Desired activities can be mimed to "kick-start" tasks. Figure/ground distinctions need to be emphasized so the person can recognize objects. Family members and care staff need help to understand the stage of dementia, which will improve their effectiveness.

TEMPORAL LOBE
Damage

FIGURE 5-4

Damage Continues: Involvement of the Temporal Lobe

The disease next attacks the *temporal lobe,* the area of the brain just beneath the temple. The temporal lobe is the center of speech and language control, and is also responsible for time awareness.

At this point in the disease process the person with Alzheimer's disease must cope with yet another devastating loss as they experience problems with communication. Communication is what makes us uniquely human—it is the way we reach out to one another, make our wishes known, and give voice to our thoughts and feelings. Once a person loses the ability to communicate she slips into a subhuman limbo and begins to lose control of her life. Others speak for her, make decisions for her, determine her needs and wishes as they see fit. The person with dementia becomes invisible.

People with temporal lobe damage demonstrate the following deficits:

- They forget names, even those of close family members.
- They have problems finding the right word to express what they mean, and may say "no" for "yes" or "purse" for "nurse" (this is called *anomia*).
- They ask questions repeatedly, seeking information they can't retain.
- They cannot string ideas together, and may lose their train of thought in mid-sentence (the phenomenon of the dangling sentence—e.g., "I would like to…" is called *abulia*). They may get up to go somewhere and forget where they are going. (All of us do this from time to time. It does not mean we have dementia!)
- They may develop *Broca's aphasia,* in which people speak haltingly or telegraphically because of difficulties in word-finding: "Doctor…going… coming…who…") or substitute a word for an entirely different one ("I don't like carburetors" rather than "I don't like cauliflower").
- They may repeat the same meaningless sound or word over and over, echo sounds *(echopraxia),* or speak gibberish or "word salad" that is difficult to understand (a symptom of *Wernicke's aphasia*): "I don't want to burn myself. I found myself. I was gone. I have to go back again. It's the same thing. I can't…figure…."
- They may have total *expressive/receptive aphasia,* in which people lose all sense of the meaning of words. Aphasia presents many problems: it may affect the production of written and spoken language, compromising both the person's ability to communicate, and the ability to acquire information from signs, messages, or notes. A person may become mute due to fear of making a mistake in speech. Language comprehension may be affected, leaving the person unable to understand what people are saying. This problem is compounded when many different people provide care in a noisy environment.

As time awareness becomes affected, the person slowly slips into a time warp. The present becomes confused; the person cannot look forward to the future; and past memories can be accessed only with help.

Seasons become meaningless. The normal cycle of the day becomes confused. People in this situation—

- repeatedly ask for assistance with time orientation, such as "Is it time yet?"; "What time is dinner?"; "Am I late for . . . ?"; "What day is it?"; "When is supper?"; "I have to get to work"; "I must get the children off to school;"
- have decreased knowledge of current events;
- can't remember personal history accurately (but may have "memory remnants");
- have impaired ability to travel or handle money; and
- begin to have problems performing complex tasks that require sequencing, use of equipment or supplies, or involvement with people (e.g., personal care activities, cooking, gardening, driving, etc.).

At this stage, the person with dementia denies that she is having problems. The following is a common scenario:

A 75-year-old wife comes in to visit her husband in a nursing home. The 80-year-old man looks at her and says, "Who are you?" or "Hello, Mother." He can't see himself as married to this elderly person, because due to loss of memory about recent times, he may think of himself as a 30- or 40-year-old!

The old man finds himself living in a time warp because memory of recent events has been destroyed. He can't be brought back to the present with prompts and reasoning, because the part of his brain that handles the sense of "the present"—his memory and awareness of time—has been destroyed and can no longer function. In his mind, he is living at some point in time in his past life. Clues to just where in time he is can be gained by listening to his conversation:

Let's suppose the man's wife is accompanied by their 30-year-old daughter. The man calls her by his wife's name. (The daughter probably looks a great deal like her mother did at 30.) The man remembers his wife at 30, but no longer remembers her at 75. The daughter looks more like the wife he remembers!

The daughter has her 10-year-old son with her. He is greeted by the elderly man who calls him by his own son's name. The boy looks like the man's son when the old man himself was 30 years old.

This time distortion is very frustrating for everyone concerned: the family members feel they've been forgotten, and the elderly man is caught up in confusion and helplessness. The entire family (including younger members) needs help to understand the effects of dementing disease. They need to learn strategies to help them connect with their husband/father/grandfather, instead of arguing with him about which year it is, or embarrassing him about his loss of memory, or not visiting because they are not recognized.

GENTLECARE Strategy

MINDTRIP is a technique whereby the professional caregiver helps the family to travel back in time to the period in time preoccupying the person with dementia, so that they may talk about pleasant news and happenings *in that time frame.*

Gentlecare uses several techniques to help families communicate with their loved ones effectively. For instance, the family is taught the MINDTRIP technique. People learn to ask, "What's the point in time that my father is talking about due to the disease process?"; and then they learn how to talk about pleasant news and events of that time period. The person experiencing dementia can join in the conversation because it involves long-term memory, which may still be intact.

I find that children, in particular, enjoy using this strategy. I compare their grandfather's behavior to that of someone from a science fiction episode who has experienced time travel. Once they have that image, they immediately relate to the effects of the disease, and take up their appropriate roles as caregivers and supporters.

For example, compare this frustrating conversation with the following conversation:

> Father: "How is the mother?"
> Daughter: "Whose mother, yours or mine?"
> Father: "The mother."
> Daughter: "Well, your mother is dead, for heaven's sake! And my mother is buried in Edmonton!"
> Father: "The mother's dead?"
> Daughter: "Of course, both our mothers are dead."
> Father (mournfully): "Nobody told me the mother was dead."

Sometimes you have to look really hard at the person with dementia and realize he or she is doing the very best they can.

Here's the same conversation using the Gentlecare Mindtrip strategy:

> Father: "How's the mother?"
> Daughter: "You are thinking of mother. She was someone special, wasn't she? Remember the wonderful pies she used to bake, and the rabbit stew?"

Gradually, by evoking old and pleasant memories, it's possible to draw people with Alzheimer's disease into conversations in which they *can* participate because the subject of the conversation does not involve damaged areas of the brain. The unhappy subject of death is avoided.

To build a prosthesis for people with these problems, caregivers need to apply superb and effective communication skills. Communicating with someone afflicted with dementia is exhausting and time-consuming, but may be one of the most potent therapies. The following are effective strategies:

- Avoid abstractions. Instead of saying, "He said...." try, "The doctor said...."
- Avoid questions. Questions imply a performance requirement in the form of a response. Due to language disintegration, this can be very frightening to the afflicted person. Instead, supply information. If it's necessary to ask questions, ask only one at a time. Always wait for the response...leave time for the response. Keep the

GLOSSARY

ABULIA   The inability to hold a thought long enough to complete an action or sentence.

AGNOSIA   The inability to recognize familiar stimuli (visual, auditory, tactile, etc.).

ANOMIA   The inability to recall the correct word or phrase to identify an object.

APHASIA   A deficit or loss of ability to express oneself by speech or writing; or to read or understand the speech of others.

APRAXIA   The inability to carry out skilled and purposeful movement—to make the body do what the mind wants it to.

ECHOLALIA   The meaningless repetition by a person of words addressed to him.

WORD SALAD   A jumble of seemingly meaningless words and phrases containing small bits of meaningful communication.

PERSEVERATION   The repetition of actions and/or sounds.

FIGURE 5-5

person with dementia talking and involved. Avoid noisy groups, malls, big family or social gatherings—the environment is too confusing. Praise the person frequently (and praise yourself).

- Use lots of non-verbal communication: hugs, kids, pets, touch, dancing, walking, hair brushing, nail care, flowers, aromas, perfume, lovely textures.
- Use the Mindtrip strategy. Family members should learn communication strategies, and staff can practice this with them.

The damage described thus far happens as Alzheimer's destroys the limbic system, the parietal lobe, and the temporal lobe during stages 1 through 4 of the disease (as described in Reisberg's Global Deterioration Scale).

Transition between Stages IV *and* V

The next period, the transition between stages IV and V, is a very stressful time for both the person with dementia and family caregivers. During this time, the afflicted person has memory loss, decreased language skills, decreased wayfinding ability, and diminished recognition of places, objects, and people. There may be also psychiatric problems, and there will likely be emotional instability.

The caregiver is likely exhausted, possibly physically ill, and probably socially isolated, anxious, and burned out. Frequently, all of these factors come together to create a crisis. It is not unusual at this point in the disease for families to decide that 24-hour care is required. The person with dementia is at this stage probably functioning at approximately the developmental level of an eight-year-old.

Damage to the Occipital Lobe

OCCIPITAL LOBE
Damage

FIGURE 5-6

As Stage V approaches, the disease moves to the back of the brain, where the occipital and parietal lobes meet. The *occipital lobe* and the *visual cortex* are the areas responsible for visual processing and visual significance. Damage in this area presents afflicted people with many problems:

- They lose their peripheral vision; they can now see only straight ahead. They will not be aware of objects or people to the side. They will not see a glass on a side table or someone sitting next to them.
- They lose the ability to look up, and their gaze is directed downward. They can miss signs or pictures or objects that are placed too high. They also tend to run into people or objects in their path.
- They lose the ability to focus on, or track, a moving object like a ball. This can be very frightening. It becomes impossible for them to watch and understand television, or identify staff members who move too quickly.
- They become very obsessive, and may repeat a motion over and over again.

- They often have the delusion that their spouse is unfaithful, or that "This is not my house."
- Their agitation increases.
- They engage in "rummaging" activity, which can be very disruptive to others but can provide them many hours of pleasing activity.
- As anxiety levels escalate, they wander occasionally about, making physical threats to people they encounter or verbal outbursts.
- They are disoriented in three spheres: time, place, and person.
- There may be personality changes, emotional upheavals, which under stress can lead to "violent behavior" or catastrophic reactions.
- There is a marked loss of willpower. Their consequent unwillingness to participate in activities may be misinterpreted as indicating poor motivation or noncompliance.
- They begin to suffer from *cognitive abulia:* they can't hold an idea long enough to complete an intended action.
- They may experience nausea or a general feeling of malaise.
- They lose the ability to read.

At this stage, the person with dementia is now functioning at approximately the developmental level of a five- to seven-year-old. To build a prosthesis for people with these problems, it is critical to reduce stress, glare, noise, and rush. It is helpful to lower pictures and important objects. Pictures should be substituted for written information. In care facilities, it is useful to remove carts and cleaning equipment from pathways. Television sets should be moved into areas where cognitively alert residents can enjoy them. Staff should be trained to slow down and converse with each person with dementia. In Gentlecare, this is called the Personal Therapy Concept. Staff should also be trained to use the Gift of Legacy concept as a means of orienting people with dementia. This concept involves everyone who comes in contact with the person afflicted giving them personal information about themselves; for instance: "Good morning, Mr. Smith. I understand you used to be the principal at Oak Street Elementary?"

Damage to the Motor Area

As the illness progresses into approximately Stage VI, damage moves from the visual cortex across the top of the brain to the motor area. The *motor cortex* is the area of the brain responsible for motor function, and damage to this area leads to the following difficulties:

MOTOR CORTEX
Damage

FIGURE 5-7

- The person has problems in initiating and following through with movements such as eating. This condition is known as *apraxia,* the inability to initiate purposeful movement to make the body do what the mind wants it to do.
- The person may experience problems with swallowing *(dysphagia).*
- Gait, posture, and motor planning are affected.
- The person has trouble getting up from a seated position because of the inability to organize body movements.
- There may be symptoms of rigidity, due to decreased amounts of the neurotransmitter dopamine, often due to prescription of neuroleptic drugs.
- The person leans to the side, leans forward, or pulls backward, shuffles, leans forward with knees bent, and has problems lifting the feet. He may exhibit *hypotonia* (muscle weakness).
- Balance is compromised.
- The person may experience *hyperkinesis* (a feeling of restlessness, with the need to move about).
- There may be muscle cramping.
- The person at this stage may show *hypermetamorphasis* (a fascination with small objects). People with hypermetamorphasis may worry at or pick at a spot or tiny object such as a design in clothing or upholstery, or eat buttons or jewelry parts.
- In later stages, the person may curl into a fetal position.

To build a prosthesis for people with these problems, caregivers must safety-proof the physical environment, getting rid of shiny, slippery surfaces, or surfaces with too much texture or pile. It helps if the afflicted person wears good footwear.

When assisting the person to walk, stand close beside and take a firm hold on the forearm for support. Never walk backwards, holding out your arms to the person. This does not afford sufficient steady support. Do not try to walk behind the person being assisted; if you cannot be seen or heard, the person may not like being touched, or held, or propelled forward.

At this stage, the use of physical restraints should be avoided. Instead, try preparing a variety of seating locations, and change from one to another during the course of the day. Limit the size of the space within which the person moves, to reduce environmental stimuli.

In Gentlecare, "soft rooms" are used for people in this stage of disease. These are small, lovely rooms with carpeting, soft furniture (often modular) with pillows, and interesting objects. Such spaces allow people to move about freely and safely, and be comforted by the ambiance.

Damage to the Occipital Region Continues

Damage to the *occipital* region continues, causing increased visual impairment. The afflicted person can now distinguish only contrasts; consequently, if caregivers wear white or pastels (the usual colors of institutional uniforms) the person has difficulty seeing them, and may resist treatment or care, especially at night. The person may not be able to distinguish a white toilet standing on a light-colored floor, and may therefore tend to use clearly defined objects (planters or dust bins) as toilets instead.

The person begins to suffer from *mind blindness,* and is unable to distinguish night from day. This results in wakefulness at night (with a need for support at that time) and also in a desire to nap during the day.

MORE OCCIPITAL LOBE
Damage

FIGURE 5-8

Damage to the Limbic System Continues

As Stage VI progresses, the limbic system, including the *hypothalamus,* is destroyed completely. The hypothalamus is the area of the brain responsible for control of temperature, thirst, and appetite. As a result—
- People may feel cold deep in their bones, or be uncomfortably hot.
- Thirst can be extreme.
- They have an enormous appetite, partly because, due to memory

MORE LIMBIC SYSTEM
Damage

FIGURE 5-9

loss, they do not remember when they last ate. Often, they will eat anything, even if the substance is toxic or disgusting, since their sense of taste and smell has been destroyed.

- They are unaware of recent events and their surroundings.
- There may be evidence of personality and emotional changes, which can cause a variety of challenging behaviors whenever the person is stressed.

To build a prosthesis for people with these problems, caregivers must develop—

- a hydration program offering the person six to eight cups of water each day. It is important to monitor liquid intake, as the affected person may require assistance with drinking.
- a means of keeping the person's body temperature at a comfortable level. It is necessary to experiment to find the appropriate room temperature and clothing needed.
- a means of monitoring food intake, due to a condition known as *pica* (a tendency to eat anything at all, including harmful substances).

PREFRONTAL AREA
Damage

FIGURE 5-10

Damage to the Prefrontal Area

As Stage VI continues, the *prefrontal* area of the brain is damaged, which causes further motor planning problems. Concurrently, damage to the visual cortex continues, and more visual changes occur. The person is affected by severe apraxia, and is unable to make the body do what they want it to, or what caregivers would like it to do. The person cannot follow directions.

Visual changes continue, and now include the problem of *visual field neglect* (inability to be aware of one side of the visual field, usually the left side). This means that at this stage the person with dementia may not be aware of food or drinks placed on one side of their food tray, or of people standing outside their field of vision.

To build a prosthesis for people with these problems, caregivers assist the person by "kick-starting" movement, and offering further help only as required. Directions must be given slowly and clearly, using mimed gestures and verbal prompts. The person's attention must be directed to the neglected side of the body, and items should be placed directly in the line of vision. At meals, the plate should be turned around so the person becomes aware of food on the neglected side.

At this point, the person is functioning at a developmental level of a child between four and five years of age.

Frontal Lobe Damage

As the disease progresses to the end of Stage VI, *frontal lobe* damage occurs. At this stage of the disease, the frontal lobe slowly ceases functioning. The critical functions of cognition (thought formation, reasoning, judgement, abstract thinking, and social consciousness) are lost.

FRONTAL LOBE
Damage

FIGURE 5-11

The disease causes the affected person to become totally focused on personal needs, no longer able to feel concern for or be aware of others. People in this stage of dementia demand instant gratification. They are uninhibited in all their actions, including sexual activity. Because memory has been lost, the afflicted person does not have the benefit of past experience, and therefore cannot anticipate the consequences of behavior. In consequence, people with dementia have diminished social judgement.

To build a prosthesis for people with these problems, caregivers must offer the kind of care given to a tiny child. They are now functioning at a developmental level equal to that of a child between two and three years of age. People at this stage should not be integrated with other client populations. Care is offered at a sensory level: touch, massage, supervised visits of children and pets, rocking, wrapping, crooning, and spiritual care.

These people must be relieved of responsibility for their actions. Both staff and family benefit from education about the effects of the disease, particularly with respect to sexual activity.

Damage to the Cerebellum

Finally, *subcortical* damage occurs. The subcortex (*hind brain*, or *cerebellum*) controls the vital involuntary body systems: the heart, lungs, diaphragm, digestive system, and some coordination and balance functions. The body begins to shut down, and death is not far off:

- The body fails to thrive, no matter what interventions are undertaken.
- The person experiences irreversible weight loss as the body metabolism burns fat. This stage is very difficult for the families who worry that the person is starving to death, and wonder if artificial feeding would help.
- The involuntary systems of the body begin to fail.
- It is not unusual for a person with Alzheimer's disease to die of a secondary infection, such as a lung or bladder infection.
- Sensory areas continue to be affected. The person will process things such as positive or negative, warm or cold, sweet or sour, dry or wet, pleasant or frightening.

CEREBELLUM
Damage

FIGURE 5-12

The person is now functioning at a developmental level equal to that of a child between the ages of 4–12 weeks and 15 months. The prosthesis at this stage consists of total care, like that one would provide for a baby. Good hydration programs, massage, wrapping, rocking, and comforting strategies are recommended.

The role of family is critical, so a good deal of effort is directed at helping the family through this stage. Family members often take comfort in being able to "do something" for their loved one: they can play music or read favorite pieces aloud such as poems and prayers. Massage and hair, hand, and foot care is soothing as well. Sometimes favorite pets are comforting.

The family needs to be supported to stay with the person as death nears. Family presence seems to provide a powerful source of comfort for the dying person at a sensory level. It is important to provide a room where the family can rest and get refreshments. A designated staff liaison person is very effective in supporting family members. Staff mem-

CORRESPONDENCE OF STAGES IN ALZHEIMER'S DISEASE TO FUNCTIONAL AGES		
Stage I Stage II	Not discernible	Functions as an adult
Stage III	Deficits in employment skills	Functions as a young adult
Stage IV	Requires help with complex tasks	8 years to adolescence
Stage V	Moderately severe dementia	5 to 7 years
Stage VI	Severe—requires assistance with self-care	24 months to 5 years
Stage VII	Very severe dementia— requires total assistance	4 to 12 weeks to 15 months

FIGURE 5-13

bers also need support at this critical time of loss. Everyone must live the reality of Alzheimer's disease, while celebrating the memory of the afflicted person.

6

Violence and Aggression: Learned Behavior

Chimera (ki-'mir-a)—*an imaginary monster compounded of incongruous parts, an illusion, fabrication of the mind, something existing only as the product of unrestrained imagination.*

Violence is the chimera of dementia. Like the fire-breathing monster of Greek mythology, violence swirls through dementia literature and practice: violence carried out by elders against one another, violence done to staff, violence acted out against families—and heartrending violence in the form of invasive practices imposed on sick, elderly people.

Why has violence become so prominent and pervasive an element in health care systems devoted to the care of the elderly? Why has attention been focused on the belligerent, angry behavior of afflicted people, rather than on the nature of the diseases or the context of care? Is elder care merely a microcosm of society as a whole, or are we in health care experiencing an aberration?

Families are aghast when they hear language that is totally out of character coming from the lips of someone they love; or when their mother or father turns on them in an ugly rage; or when they hear their loved ones described as aggressive or dangerous by professional staff.

It is claimed that violence perpetuated by elderly people against staff is increasing in incidence and severity. A very large part of the agenda of elder care concerns itself with the management of violent be-havior. Texts, journals, courses, behavioral strategies, investigating committees, labor agreements, specialized equipment, and repressive sanctions have developed as a result of this preoccupa-tion. In some cases, the residential units for people with dementia are referred to as "behavior wards," "locked units," or "management areas," as if the environment were dedicated to containing some dangerous animal. The myth that violence is an inevitable outcome of de-mentia has flourished to the point where more attention is invested in documenting perceived abusive behavior than in developing care programs to prevent it. Based on the perception that people with dementia are dangerous or violent, a locked area becomes a "lockdown," and the people who live within it are imprisoned by that percep-tion, rather than by the limitations of their illness.

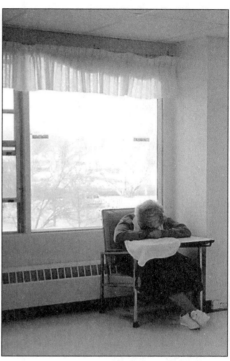

Isolation and immobilization contribute to frustration, fear, and aggression.

I FOUND A MAN IN HIS LATE 50s *lying flat on his back in a reclined geriatric chair. My attention was drawn to him because beside the chair was an IV pole— somewhat unusual equipment for a dementia care area! His wrists were manacled to the chair at his sides, as were his ankles. A feeding tube led out of his stomach and he was catheterized. When I leaned close to him he said, "Please help me die."*

I asked the staff why such extreme measures had been taken. I learned that the man was in the early stages of Alzheimer's disease. He was confused and angry about his hospitalization, and deter-mined to go to his construction company site. He had made an at-tempt to do so, and was physically restrained and returned to his room, where, in frustration, he lashed out at staff members. They called for backup, and his response was to fight even harder. Staff members were injured in the fracas. The restraint, feeding, and elim-ination measures had been applied as a result of his resistance.

Unfamiliar environments filled with glare, rush, and strangers create terror.

Why the Violence?

As we have seen, dementing illnesses such as Alzheimer's disease assail the emotional centers of control during the earliest stages of the disease. As damage continues, the ability to interpret external stimuli, to tolerate stress, communicate, and finally to use reason and judgement is lost. From the onset of Alzheimer's disease, afflicted people lose the ability to manage life's challenges. The emotional controls that healthy people take for granted are absent. The social mores that direct our lives are eroded. The cognitive process that permits us to figure out solutions to problems or deal with other people has been destroyed. People who can no longer handle ordinary situations become frightened.

Then we place these terrified people into psychiatric hospitals, units for the physically disabled, chronic care institutions, or "holding units" in medical/surgical facilities. Should we be surprised when they react aggressively to the stress inherent in those situations? Should we, in fact, categorize their behavior as aggression at all, or should we understand that in their fear and frustration, they react with the only behavior available to them: resistance?

Resistance can easily evolve into aggression. Even the tiniest, mildest old lady will fight like a tiger if she perceives herself to be cornered and in danger. And if such a person feels repeatedly threatened by the stresses of her surroundings, her normal response whenever she encounters the same stresses may well be to become assaultive. Let us try to imagine how she feels.

How would you feel if you were sitting in your room and a complete stranger of the opposite sex came up to insist that you get undressed and have a bath in a public room? How would you respond if someone unknown woke you up at night and insisted that you go to the bathroom accompanied by that person? What would you do if you found yourself locked in a strange place with dozens of other sick people, and were told that this was your home? Of course you would be enraged in any of these situations and the resistance that they provoke begins to sound appropriate, given the circumstances!

Turning Things Around

I was once asked to work with two men who were "violent" at wake-up time each morning. Upon investigation, I found that staff on the evening shift awakened the people with dementia at 4:30 every morning, and did their grooming and dressing.

"Why so early?" I inquired.

"Oh, to get them ready."

"Ready for what?!"

"Well, just ready."

It turned out that this practice gave the day staff an early start on the day's work, making it possible to have everyone ready for breakfast at 7:30 A.M. The two gentlemen in question clearly resisted being awakened from a deep sleep, and proceeded to swear at and hit anyone who tried to force them to get up. Medication had been prescribed to control the violent behavior.

We decided to try a different strategy: let them sleep in and wake-up naturally. This notion initially met with a great deal of resistance:

"They'll sleep all day."

"We'll never get our work done."

"They'll miss breakfast."

As it turned out, when staff went about their work but left the two men to sleep in, they woke up naturally around 7:00 A.M., were able to manage most of their own grooming, and were among the first to show up in the dining room.

A choice all of us would like to exercise!

The Gentlecare strategy of choice in this case was to allow a flexible routine around wake-up and meal times. Setting that strategy in place involved—

- communicating with all staff about the implications of the new plan;

- assessing the impact of change on each department or work group;
- planning for any necessary schedule changes, and finding solutions for any problems such changes might create;
- ensuring that all staff knew what to do and what not to do in the new circumstances;
- developing alternate menus and eating locations;
- trying out the plan;
- evaluating results;
- identifying and making any necessary changes to the plan; and finally
- celebrating the changes in functioning!

It is not because things are difficult that we do not dare. It is because we do not dare that they are difficult.

—SENECA

The institution where those two gentlemen live has now implemented the "relaxed breakfast" for all residents. When the idea of doing so was first broached, staff in many areas expressed great anxiety:

"How will everything get done on time?"

"How will we keep track of medications?"

"Will we have to reschedule activities?"

Three weeks after implementing the new flexible routines, staff comments sounded like this:

"This is great!"

"The dining room is operating very well; in fact, clean-up is happening a few minutes earlier than usual!"

"The residents are calmer."

"Residents are often awake and usually getting ready on their own by the time we get there to help them."

As well, one gentleman who previously required total care now manages his own self-care and is on a walking program. One lady who had always required total care now sleeps in and gets her own toast and coffee in the dayroom.

Comments from the residents were also positive:

"I love being able to snuggle back into bed for a while before breakfast."

"I'm much more relaxed and I sleep better knowing I don't have to get up."

"I love having toast and tea when I'm properly awake. I love mornings now!"

Buoyed by the positive results, staff members at the facility are eager to try new ways of delivering care. They are relaxed, proud of their accomplishments, and find they can do the same amount of work in a shorter period of time than was previously required. Residents are functioning at a higher level of competency, and everyone feels pleased.

It should be noted that these changes happened because everyone decided to make them happen.

Violence does not equal dementia. Violence results from the effects of dementia.

The Context of Violence

Linear and Lateral Thinking

Violence must be considered within the context of issues such as—

- the nature of the person's disease;
- the extent of dysfunction;
- the level of stress/fatigue/anxiety of all parties;
- the degree to which the person understands what's being done to him;
- the number of people involved;
- staff attitudes and approaches; and
- the environmental context.

Try substituting the word terror for aggression.

Our current health care system is *linear*. It is structured to respond to crisis defensively, rather than to understand and avoid crises. For example, suppose the problem was that a person with dementia struck out at a caregiver during personal care. A caregiver using a linear approach to the problem would document the incident, and give the person a psychoactive medication to calm him down. The person would then become comatose, and would thus be easier to groom and dress.

A linear care plan acts quickly and dramatically, but has terrible long-term effects. Facing the same problem, a caregiver using *lateral* thinking would—

- ask why the patient had struck out;
- want to know who was involved in the interaction;
- find out what was going on in the environment;
- ask if the person understood the procedure;
- consider the necessity for the procedure;
- ask if the person had received an "energy boost" (a drink or some food) before undertaking the task;
- want to know if the person had been allowed to rest between stages of the task;
- ask whether a different plan of approach had been tried, and tried again; and
- ask if different people had tried to help.

This kind of plan takes longer to implement, but it solves the problem instead of masking it, and prevents the development of long-range, costly problems. However, non-linear or system thinking is anything but easy. It involves a real commitment on the part of everyone offering care to understand and empathize with the person, rather than judge or condemn. It comes from a place of love—not fear.

Some will argue that non-linear planning is too time-consuming, but experience shows that in the long run, this is simply not true. Such strategies help the afflicted person to improve function; they support family caregivers, make it easier for professional caregivers, and make care itself less expensive.

ONCE UPON A TIME *I filmed a 56-year-old man who had Alzheimer's disease. He had been a very successful business executive, and was part of a lovely family. The disease had tragically devastated large portions of his speech centers, but with support and care, the essential human being behind the disease could be reached. During the course of the disease, this man reacted violently to stress in his environment, and was hospitalized.*

Thirteen months later I saw this same man again. Perceived as dangerous and agitated, he was receiving large doses of antipsychotic medication. He was restrained in a geriatric chair. His head hung on

Staff in one facility wore lapel buttons that read: "Have you been hurt today?"

It is wonderful what a different view we take of the same event four and twenty hours after it has happened.

—SIDNEY SMITH, ENGLISH CLERGYMAN 1771

his chest. He was drooling and asleep. He was "too ill" to participate in any activity.

I sat and talked with him about his part in the film we had done together. I told him that the interview he did with me had helped people like himself all across the country. Thinking he was asleep, I got up to leave, but realized he was crying. He said, very carefully, very painfully, "I tried . . . we tried, Moyra."

Supporters of linear or closed systems look at such a person and see a middle-aged, physically fit man, agitated and anxious. They perceive danger. They know their perception is real, because in fact, under stress this person had been violent. Chemical restraint is the obvious, easiest, fastest, and most widely practiced response to his behavior. Linear thinking localizes the problem in the person with dementia. The problem is "fixed" by altering his ability to function. But is it?

This is an example of empty hand syndrome— people engaged in no activity, often for up to 12 hours each day.

Supporters of a participatory system (or lateral approach) look at the same person and see someone whose dynamic, independent personality has been severely stressed by being placed in an environment that— from his perspective—tried to take control of his life. Supporters of such a participatory approach would find the root of the problem in the poor fit between the individual's personality/life experience and the environment in which he found himself. They would seek to resolve the problem by assessing the person's functional level and finding safe areas of personal autonomy for him; by making sure he understood why certain procedures were necessary; by relaxing schedules and rules where possible; and by changing other social and environmental factors to support his personality and remaining skills.

The bottom line in eliminating the sense of violence surrounding dementia is that if change is to occur, the change must happen within the agents of the system. We must change the system of health care because the person with dementia can't.

There are four common elements in the present model of dementia care that magnify the phenomenon of violent behavior. All four also contribute to accelerated dysfunction, excessive disability, and rising health care costs. They are: externalizing the problem; misuse of medication; the power of inappropriate language to shape inappropriate action; and the misuse of restraint. Each of these elements is discussed below.

Externalizing the Problem

Man did not weave the web of life, he is merely a strand in it. Whatever he does to the web, he does to himself.

—CHIEF SEATTLE

The assumption in most care facilities is that violence is an expected and enduring aspect of the workplace. If you work with people who have Alzheimer's disease, chances are you will get punched or kicked or bitten. Consequently, staff members take turns or draw lots to see who is unlucky enough to have to "do" Mr. X today. Staff members work in pairs (or three- or five-person teams) to give Mr. X a bath or to change his clothes.

Furthermore, the approach to violence in health care traditionally has not been focused on seeking the reasons for its occurrence, but rather on finding ways to manage it or reduce the impact of assaults on staff. In current practice, surveys and staff abuse recording tools focus on such issues as—

- staff fitness;
- effective alarm systems;
- patients' history of assault;
- identifying potentially assaultive behavior toward each staff member;
- procedures for reporting assaults to the administration and to the police;
- legal penalties;
- support for assaulted staff;
- restraint procedures;
- job satisfaction issues; and
- physical/mental exhaustion of staff.

But, as the philosopher Wheeler observed, to understand anything in nature we must cross out the old word *observer* and put in place the new word *participant*. To comment on a person's behavior, therefore, is really to comment on the nature of one's own interaction with the sick person. A report of violence is in itself an admission of failure on our part as caregivers to meet one or more of the specific needs of a person in our care, whether that need is for more information, a slower pace, calm and quiet, or a hug.

> *From physics to psychology, every department of science is realizing more and more that to observe the world is to participate in it, and that as frustrating as this may first seem to be, it is the most important clue to all further knowledge.*
>
> —ALLAN BATES

At the same time, it must be recognized that failure to meet the needs of people with dementia does not mean that caregivers are stupid, cruel, or uncaring. It simply means that they must try something else, or try one more time. We must try to understand the disease more clearly; try to put ourselves in the other person's shoes; try talking about the problem with another caregiver or the person's spouse. There is something we must do differently. We must find out what that something is and do it differently until the person with dementia is comfortable.

Violence can't be isolated from its context, or from ourselves as participants in the context. Staff abuse is not a patient problem—it is a system problem. To reduce the violence shown by persons with dementia, we must dare to examine and understand the whole system that operates where we work. Conscious participation is necessary. We must not only understand ourselves, but also the systems we create and perpetuate. We must evaluate our actions and the systems we operate, in relation to those who need our help. Jung referred to this process as ac-

Please listen carefully, and try to hear what
I am not saying
what I would like to be able to say.
What for survival, I need
to say, but I can't say.
Each time you are kind,
and gentle, and encouraging,
Each time you try to understand because you really care,
My heart grows wings
very feeble wings, but wings.
I want you to know how
important
you are to me.
Who am I?
You may wonder.
I am someone you know very well
For I am every man you meet
I am every woman.
I am you.

—Author Unknown

Sometimes a shoulder to lean on comes in handy.

ceptance. We cannot change anything unless we accept it. Condemnation does not liberate us from our problems, it only creates new ones.

In the example on page 61, we see violence exchanged for dependency. Acceptance, on the other hand, opens and releases our creativity to find new solutions, to find and help the person who still exists behind the disease.

Misuse of Medication

In many care facilities, aggressive behavior is controlled by the widespread use of chemical substances that were designed for other purposes: antipsychotics, antidepressants, and anti-anxiety/hypnotic drugs. People with dementing illness are sedated with these medications after catastrophic behavior has occurred, or in anticipation of future violence.

The use of drugs to restrain a person with dementia is perhaps the most serious chemical threat to safety and well-being in the long-term care environment—though that threat to safety is often unconscious and unintended.

I REMEMBER DISCUSSING the situation of a tiny woman patient. She had hit out at a staff member who had approached her abruptly from the side (by his own admission). The woman had been given Ativan, to quiet her down. That morning she hung in her restraint vest in her wheelchair in deep sleep. After lunch she was finally put to bed, as no one had been able to wake her. Just before dinner, I chanced by her room and found her still asleep.

When I inquired about her, I discovered that the afternoon staff, upon reading about the violent incident of the previous day, had given her another prescription of Ativan "as a preventive measure." It was another two days before this woman was able to eat her food by herself.

The principal strategy of quality dementia care is to assess and maintain levels of function not yet destroyed by disease. When demented people are given medication for purposes other than prescribed treatment, vital remaining functions are blotted out—not by the disease, but by medical intervention. This results in the person feeling more confused, frustrated, and vulnerable than ever, and leads inevitably to an escalation of belligerence and terror.

Medication used for restraint has a multitude of harmful effects on elderly people:
- loss of personal volition
- confusion
- heart rate change
- depression
- tardive dyskinesia
- agitation

- bladder problems
- sedation
- postural hypotension
- anxiety
- slurred speech;
- stiffness

The most important consideration for appropriate psychoactive medication usage is whether any drug is needed at all.

—JAMES W. COOPER, UNIV. OF GEORGIA NURSING HOMES

IT MUST BE EMPHASIZED THAT THE ABOVE COMMENTS REFER TO MEDICATION USED FOR RESTRAINT PURPOSES ONLY, NOT TO DRUGS USED HONESTLY AS TREATMENT MODALITIES.

It should be understood by everyone who cares about people with dementia that while there have been some encouraging preliminary results reported on drugs that help somewhat in early stage dementia only, no drug in current use ameliorates the effects of dementia. Many drugs, in fact, exacerbate the effects of Alzheimer's disease or related dementias. Nevertheless, medication is often given in the guise of treatment to calm the person down, to reduce anxiety or catastrophic behavior, or to reduce violence.

Families generally know very little about pharmaceutical treatment, and are reluctant to question the use of medication to control behavior. Many believe they cannot question the prescription of psychotropic (mood altering) medication. And yet families are frontline advocates; they must become informed and courageous enough to be able to ask: How is this drug going to change the course of dementia in my family member? Sometimes medications prescribed for other medical conditions suffered by persons with dementia can be harmful too. This is especially true if the side effects of the prescription are attributed to dementia, rather than to the drugs being given. This issue is a factor in a significant number of cases when prescriptions are not reviewed regularly nor adjusted according to the person's current health status.

HE LAY CURLED UP *on his side sleeping soundly, and gave no response as his wife gently touched his hair and spoke to him. His caregivers reported that he slept most of the time and was very resistant to*

IMPASSE

I placed my darling in a nursing home
With a special ward for folk like he.
He was welcomed and we both responded thankfully!
We felt a part of this community: it seemed a caring place.
On the ninth day my love was expelled
As "dangerous to residents and staff."
They notified me that he had been in restraints:
He was not wanted there! I was aghast!
Another place made room for him somehow to my relief:
Otherwise he would have been sent to a mental hospital!
I later found he had been over-medicated the last three days
With drugs that crazy him. For me it was disaster!
How could they ignore me, his caregiver
And the hospital staff who had known him for years?
A nursing home must be a caring place:
Its staff must have an endless store of empathy and love,
Plus training in "no restraints and minimal medication"
Techniques—that experts now espouse.
All who would care for the Alzheimer's victim must share
A true acceptance of this unique person who has dementia.
Only then can we treat him as we would want for ourselves.
A huge compelling and complex prescription—but possible!
For my love I need a caring place that loves enough
To ignore restraints and drugs—so over-used
One that can accept serenely
The fear and anger and confusion
That can occur in any Alzheimer's victim—
Where can I find this place in our imperfect world?

—Gil Ludeman

personal care. When we reviewed his care plan, I learned that he suffered from Parkinson's disease and took five medications daily for that disease.

This therapy plan had been developed several years ago when he weighed 150 lbs. and was very active. His current weight had slipped to a point that concerned everyone, and he was involved in almost no physical activity.

It was suggested that his medication be reviewed in terms of his current health status. As a result, three medications given for Parkinson's disease were discontinued. To date there have been significant—even remarkable—changes in his level of functioning. He is now able to sit up and feed himself, enjoy his wife's visits, go out for drives, and visit his home. Nothing changed in this man's dementia or Parkinson's disease. Only his medical treatment was altered.

Use of psychotropic medication in dementia care should be considered an absolute last line of defense, to be used only after every other conceivable intervention has been tried and failed, and preferably not then either.

Inappropriate Language Shapes Inappropriate Action

Language is not neutral—it plays an active part in shaping what we think of things and people. A large part of the difficulty we have in accepting the person with dementia is caused by the way language is used in our health care system.

LANGUAGE VERSUS EXPERIENCE

The relationship between language and experience is often misunderstood. Language actually defines experience for us by reason of its formal completeness, and because of our unconscious projection of its implicit expectations into the field of experience.

—Edward Sapir,
Conceptual Categories in Primitive Languages

Labels abound in dementia care, and most of them are negative: dirty old man, spitter, aggressive, feeder, problem patient, and vegetative are only a few examples. Labels pin behavior on individuals, irrespective of context or the role of others. Placing a negative label on someone suggests that the labeled individual is acting with malicious intent, premeditation, and/or in order to control the behavior of others. Careful study of the pathology of dementing illnesses demonstrates the impossibility of any of those intentions.

The language we use has the power to change the emotional intent of what we say. For example, the Latin prefix *dis-* means apart, asunder, away, or having a negative or reversing force. It is used in the construction of such common words as disability, disbelief, dishearten, or dislike. In the vocabulary of dementia care, *dis-* appears in such words as disoriented or dysfunctional. Disorient, for example, means to cause to lose one's way (the strange streets disoriented him); to confuse by removing or obscuring something that has guided the person, group, or culture such as customs or moral standards (society has been disoriented by changing values); and in psychiatry, to cause to lose perception of time, place, or one's personal identity. The use of the word disorient clearly describes the terror and confusion of old people as their cognitive ability slowly and inexorably declines.

The Latin prefix *mal-*, on the other hand, means bad, wrongful, ill. It is commonly used in such words as malfunction, malcontent, maladroit, and maladjusted. In dementia care, a new word has been coined (not found in the dictionary): *maloriented*. This word is used to describe people who are oriented but not happily so, people who are "unhappy" because they need to resolve past emotional issues and unresolved conflicts. When such made-up language is used to describe elders who experience psychiatric and/or dementing illnesses, the implication is that it is their responsibility to change their bad behavior, and therefore that the onus to do so rests with them. Language imposes this burden on those who have little or no control over their behavior.

People afflicted with a dementing illness can never be reoriented to time, place, or person, because of the progressive nature of their disease. With help, their state of disorientation can be supported, and its

If thought corrupts language, language also corrupts thought.

—GEORGE ORWELL

Sticks and stones are hard on bones Aimed with an angry art: Words can sting like anything And silence breaks the heart.

—ANONYMOUS

side effects can be ameliorated. With support, a person with dementing disease will be less fearful, less frustrated, less confused, and less angry, but not less disoriented.

The language we use shapes the way we think about, approach, plan for, and ultimately care for people with dementia. And not only is our thinking influenced by these labels—so is the thinking of everyone to whom we talk about the person with dementia. Spouses frequently talk to me about their violent husbands. When I ask, "What gives you the idea that your husband is violent?" they reply, "I was told he was." When I ask what their own impression is, they often say, "You know, Moyra, my husband never ever acted this way until he got sick. It's so unlike him." Labels impede effective dementia care—and they are cruel.

Restraint as a Metaphor for Failure

The use of restraint on elderly people living in health care facilities is so pervasive that it cries out to be examined: What is the rationale for this phenomenon?

There has been a great reluctance on the part of policy makers in the care of the elderly to acknowledge and address the issue of cognitive impairment in those in residential care facilities. Traditionally, people living in facilities have been expected to understand the procedures associated with illness and care, and comply with staff requests—in fact, to be appreciative of their services. As the population of residential care facilities has changed, however, more and more of those in care are people who lack the reasoning and judgement to accept care. Many are, in fact, resistant to care and unwilling to comply with staff directions.

Rather than attempting to understand the needs of such people and adapt to them, health care services have opted to make cognitively impaired elderly people comply with expected behavioral norms—even though such people lack the cognitive ability to do so!

In some large psychiatric hospitals, restraint devices are part of the daily linen distribution: all patients are restrained, as part of the program. When complaints are received in such situations, staff is bewil-

POSTURE IN RESTRAINT-RELATED DEATHS

Drawings by Robert English, adapted from originals by Elizabeth Dempsey. Used with permission of Biomedical Graphic Communication Department at the University of Minnesota, from *The Gerontologist,* Vol. 32, No. 6, 762–766, December 1992.

FIGURE 6-1

 77   CHAPTER SIX

dered: the use of restraints has become so normal that they don't understand what the fuss is all about.

What's the easiest way to ensure that mobile, resistant, non-compliant people suffering from dementing illnesses conform to norms of behavior? The answer is the use of restraints—physical, chemical, environmental, and psychological. Tying up, drugging, and threatening vulnerable elderly people—under the guise of providing health care—truly represents the ultimate failure of the system. To change such practices, we must understand what they are and their consequences, and we must create alternatives.

Physical Restraints

A physical restraint is any physical or mechanical device, material, or equipment adjacent to the person's body that restricts movement or normal function of the body, and which the individual cannot remove. Examples of physical restraints are—

- vests or shirts
- wrist straps
- ankle cuffs
- sheets
- groin/pelvic straps
- abdominal belts
- wheelchairs
- wall hooks
- lock-down food trays
- mitts
- bed tables
- bed rails
- "Geri-chairs" (geriatric chairs, recliners)
- elevated chairs/soft chairs, such as bean bag chairs
- "paired cuffing" to another person

Environmental Restraints

An environmental restraint is any structure or impediment which is built into the environment in order to limit or restrict personal mobility and the exercise of will. Examples of environmental restraints are—

- maze/look-alike corridors
- circular corridors
- seclusion rooms
- isolation
- shiny floors
- fences
- large open spaces
- alarm systems
- doors, locked doors, and alarmed doors

```
┌─────────────────────────────────────────────────────────┐
│            EFFECTS OF MEDICATION USED                    │
│             FOR RESTRAINT PURPOSES                       │
│                                                          │
│   • confusion              • depression                  │
│   • slurred speech         • agitation                   │
│   • bladder problems       • blurred vision              │
│   • sedation               • constipation                │
│   • dizziness              • drooling/dry mouth           │
│   • heart rate change      • stiffness                   │
│   • tardive dyskinesia (involuntary movement)            │
│   • postural hypotension (inability to maintain body posture) │
│   • anxiety                                              │
│   • and more...                                          │
└─────────────────────────────────────────────────────────┘
```

FIGURE 6-2

- confusing areas, such as a complicated route to the outdoors
- sensors on beds or chairs attached to people and triggered when they move

Chemical Restraints

Chemical restraints are any medications given to control mood, mental status, or behavior, that have no therapeutic benefit. Such restraints include—
- mood-altering medication
- psychoactive drugs
- tranquilizers and sedatives

Psychological Restraints

Psychological restraints are threats or verbal requirements that restrict a person's freedom of movement or will. These include—
- warnings
- threats
- withdrawal of privileges
- requests (from a position of power)

I VISITED A VERY QUIET *dementia unit some years ago. Every single person sat quietly in their chair. No one except staff moved around the unit. This was so unusual that at first I suspected chemical restraint, but a review of the charts indicated only normal use of medication. As I passed a bedroom a tiny lady who had been peering out scuttled back to the chair beside her bed. When I went to talk to her she appeared very anxious and frightened, and asked, "Am I going to be allowed to come out today?"*

Restraints may be imposed for purposes of discipline, for convenience, or because of low staffing levels. They in no way contribute to the treatment or performance ability of a person with dementia. A number of restraints may be used in combination, compounding the risk of damage to people.

Safety Devices versus Restraints

Physical restraints should be clearly differentiated from safety devices. Restraints are used to restrict movement. Safety or rehabilitative devices, on the other hand, enhance the person's functional ability and safety. Examples of safety devices are padded lap belts on wheelchairs that allow the person to move about safely and independently; and a chest harness that allows a person with weak back muscles or postural dysfunction to remain upright in a functional position. Such devices are individually prescribed, and adapted to the individual's specific requirements. They are checked regularly, and adjusted as the person's condition changes. Most improve the person's level of function and are welcomed by the person wearing them.

On occasion, family members actually request the use of restraints, or support staff members in using restraints—usually because they are worried about fractures, or because they are afraid that if their family member doesn't comply with regulations, he will be discharged or transferred to a psychiatric institution.

Common Arguments for the Use of Restraint

The use of restraint as a means of managing people with dementia, however, is not without its proponents. Many of the arguments used to

DESTRUCTIVE EFFECTS
OF RESTRAINTS

- loss of personal freedom and will
- loss of bone mass, weakened bone stucture
- decrease in muscle function/strength/mass
- deterioration of skin tissue, ulcers, pressure sores
- lower extremity swelling
- changes in metabolism
- loss of balance, falls
- increase in incontinence and elimination problems
- loss of independent toileting
- sensory deprivation
- psychiatric disorders
- depressed psychological status
- decrease in social behavior/interaction
- increased problems with sleep patterns
- gastrointestinal stress
- decreased interest in eating
- loss of energy
- increased dependency, learned helplessness
- emotional disorders, withdrawal
- increased agitation
- angry, belligerent or combative behavior
- stress to staff, families, others
- injuries
- muscle contractions
- death

FIGURE 6-3

support restraint use essentially focus on organizational issues. It is argued that restraints—

- provide answers to safety concerns;
- can compensate for inadequate numbers or levels of staff;
- minimize fear of liability due to falls;
- compensate for lack of adequate or appropriate environments;
- substitute for lack of secure perimeters in buildings, such as fences and alarmed doors;

- solve the problems that arise when people with different levels of cognitive functioning share accommodations; and
- prevent confrontation between afflicted people or between people and staff, which leave bruises and therefore raise questions of abuse.

The only thing necessary for evil to triumph is for good men to do nothing.

—EDMOND BURKE

A Word on Wheelchairs

Wheelchairs are a North American disease! Elderly people, especially those living within institutions, often spend their lives in wheelchairs.

Wheelchairs were originally designed as necessary equipment for seriously paralyzed or paraplegic patients. Eventually, people began to use them to move elderly people quickly from point A to point B. The problem arises when wheelchairs become an elderly person's home. As a rule, wheelchairs do not have good seating: the person's spine is not supported, and over time, this causes acute discomfort and pain. Elderly people often lack the muscle strength to change or adjust their sitting position—especially if a restraint device is used in combination with a wheelchair.

Wheelchairs have evolved into restraints.

Wheelchairs are often placed in front of blaring television sets, grouped in front of nursing stations, or lined up in busy hallways—with the ostensible objective of stimulating their occupants. Elderly people only rarely have the necessary muscle power to move themselves to a more comfortable, quiet location. Thus, ironically, a rehabilitative device designed to improve function and mobility has evolved into a restraint, and in fact is often the cause of dysfunction.

If a wheelchair is to act as a prosthetic device, it should be individually designed to meet a person's needs. Wheelchairs are not interchangeable! If a wheelchair is assigned, it should be carefully prescribed in terms of size, design, seating, and adaptations by a professional staff member knowledgeable in this field. Beware of wide chairs that provide no support for tiny women, or regular or narrow chairs that pinch or rub larger men. Wheelchairs should always provide support for the legs and feet.

Avoid the use of plexiglass tables with people experiencing dementia. It is very disconcerting to have an obstacle that cannot be properly perceived (a clear table) between the upper and lower part of one's body. Similarly, objects that float without obvious support are very confusing. Avoid attaching so-called sensory stimulating objects such as busy boards to table tops on a permanent basis.

THE FOLLOWING ARE SOME SUGGESTIONS FOR STRATEGIES
THAT CAN BE USED AS ALTERNATIVES TO RESTRAINT:

Do unto others as if you were the other.

- Assessment of the person with dementia by an interdisciplinary team, including the family, identifies the person's strengths and weaknesses as well as lifelong habits, daily routines, attitudes, memory capability, disease status, activity interests, and family dynamics. Information on the medical profile is critical.

- Assessment is ongoing. Persons with dementia require an individualized care plan that guides everyone in their contact with the affected person. Such a care plan must be communicated to everyone—all staff, family, volunteers, and support people.

- The care plan includes direction for approaches to the person, communication requirements, ideas for meaningful activity, ways to support the family structure, assistance necessary for management of self-care, spiritual requirements, movement programs, and any special environmental requirements.

- Environmental adaptation includes silent alarms; secured perimeters; enhanced lighting; reduced glare; comfortable furniture; indoor/outdoor access; effective signage and wayfinding cues; interesting objects/points of interest; warm, mid-range colors, especially in staff clothing; effective figure/ground contrast; small social spaces free of noise and confusion; normal, home-like ambiance; and reduced use of alarms, announcement systems, and call bells.

- Attention is given to physical needs such as hunger, thirst, movement, toileting, pain, cold, and heat.

- Attention is given to psychological needs such as fear, anxiety, loneliness, lack of support, hallucinations, delusions, confusion, disorientation, and memory loss.
- Staffing and family/volunteer levels are appropriate to the needs of people with dementia, throughout a complete 24-hour period, as is the case with any other medical specialty.
- There is flexibility in routines and schedules to allow for the progress of disease and personal needs, reduction of stress, rush, and schedule rigidity in favor of performance, activity, and interaction.
- In acute care settings, staff are trained in the care of people with dementia.
- In medical situations where intravenous equipment, dressings, or other medical material is required, it is helpful to organize teams of family members and volunteers to sit with the person with dementia through the crisis. Practices similar to those used in palliative care are most effective.
- "Soft" or "comfort" rooms which are secured should be available for people who wake during the night. Mattresses or beds low to the floor help eliminate the need for restraint.
- Development of programs and environments that support rather than challenge vulnerable individuals also help eliminate the need for restraint. These include points of interest; interesting objects, things to touch, to do; familiar, relevant activities that focus on one step, repetitive actions using old memory and former skills; focus on movement such as walking indoors and outdoors, dancing, work activity, use of volunteers, students, young people, families to assist with walking (all movement should be charted); relaxation and stress-reducing activities such as children's visits/pets, massage/bathing/manicures, one-on-one visiting; socialization programs in tiny groups of one to three people that promote fun, competency, former life activities, family connections; family conversations and specific music, or prayers, stories, etc. on tape, using Walkman or small sound systems; areas designed indoors and outdoors for safe movement; and all staff, volunteers and

families engage in validation, reminiscing and general family communication.

It is important to note that many people feel these ideas are idealistic or unrealistic in the economic climate of today's health care system. Nevertheless, it should be stressed that there are facilities all over North America and Europe that are restraint-free and practice this type of prosthetic care successfully with no increase in funding. The secret to the elimination of all types of restraint in the elderly is simple: individualized therapeutic care.

The philosophy of Gentlecare is one we can all embrace with ease when afflicted people are compliant and co-operative. It is easy to care for, respect, give control to, or communicate with the archetypal elderly man and woman: those who enjoy our company, are appreciative of

Dementia is the ultimate restraint.

The Dutch door is one of the least harmful restraint measures that allows full movement within a restricted area, and facilitates removal of a person in case of fire or emergency. This comfortable safe space allows people who can't ambulate safely to move and exercise.

FIGURE 6-4

Bed adaptation courtesy of Riverview Care Center, Washington, U.S.A.

FIGURE 6-5

service, and whose faces light up when they see us coming. It is easy to care for people when nothing is required of us except to move through a routine task that makes no demands on our cognition or creativity.

The hard part comes when we are required to honor our philosophical ideals when we are working with those who, because of illness, neither appreciate nor agree to our presence in their life. When the people we care for are resistant or show catastrophic behavior, then it becomes all too easy to forget our high-minded resolve and succumb to the seduction of old practices. It becomes easier to reach for chemical restraint than to talk the person out of distress; easier to transfer them out of our jurisdiction; easier to see the person as dangerous or violent, or someone so unpleasant as to be undeserving of our care and attention.

In those circumstances, eliminating undesirable behaviors and approaches becomes more difficult. And when inappropriate practices such as the use of restraint on elderly persons are entrenched in the system of health care, the task becomes monumental. For example, decision-making about the use of restraint can be beyond the control of individual caregivers, as it is almost always ordered by a physician, based on the information given him by care providers.

Caregivers correctly say the system has to change, because we can't do it alone. And that's true—but we are part of the system, and we can take part in changing the attitudes, assumptions, language, and approaches that underlie and support the use of restraint.

Ethical and Legal Issues

The practice of using restraints in dementia care facilities is increasingly coming under public scrutiny because it raises complex ethical and legal questions. For example, restraints are most often used on elderly persons, many of whom cannot express opinions due to cognitive impairment. But all persons, regardless of age, have the right to be free of physical and chemical restraint and (within reasonable limits) to enjoy autonomy, regardless of their level of cognition.

Restraint of any kind can be applied only on a medical order from a physician. When such orders are imposed for purposes of convenience, rather than because they are required to treat medical symptoms, the act calls into question the *Hippocratic oath* which commits a physician to do no harm.

As concern regarding the use of physical and chemical restraint increases, and the practices of applying such restraint come under regulation, a word of caution is necessary. It is far easier to disguise drug therapy as a medical strategy than it is to claim that physical restraint is a medical necessity. We must therefore all be vigilant in seeing that there is no further proliferation in the use of mood-altering drugs to control behavior in the elderly. We must also see that the use of psychologically punitive tactics does not escalate.

Family caregivers are often uninformed, misinformed, frightened, or simply not sufficiently assertive to advocate on behalf of their family members. They often feel, and are encouraged to feel, that there is no alternative to the use of restraint. But there is! Working together, we can ensure that elderly persons become truly liberated from restraint of any kind. Health care practitioners and family carers all over the world are beginning to say, "The time has come for change!"

GENTLECARE 12-POINT ACTION PLAN FOR ELIMINATING USE OF RESTRAINTS FOR PERSONS WITH DEMENTING ILLNESS

1. EDUCATE ALL STAFF and family caregivers in the process of dementing illness, the behavior caused by the disease process, and the effects of chemical and physical restraint.

2. REVIEW THE LIVING SPACE of the person with dementia. Create a safe, secure, comfortable area, however small, in which the person can move about freely.

3. REVIEW YOUR PROGRAMS to ensure that there are interesting, beautiful objects available for the person with dementia to touch, move, enjoy, and interact with. Use music, pets, books, pictures, flowers, old jewelry, stuffed toys, purses, briefcases, mops, dusters, brooms, rummage opportunities, pillows, afghans, cards, folding towels, different sized boxes, etc. Make the environment feel like home.

4. ASSESS ONE PERSON AT A TIME—review all medication. Consider discontinuing any medication that does not have a therapeutic effect on the person receiving it. Consider dosage, length of time administered, reasons for giving each medication, circumstances under which medication was given or order requested, and by whom it was requested. Review circumstances before medication use and effects of medication on the person's level of function for at least two days following use of the medication. Review patterns of staff practice. Who uses medication? Who uses alternate strategies? Record findings.

5. ONE PERSON AT A TIME—review type or combination of physical restraint being used. Review length of time person is under restraint. Review practice of adjusting or checking restraint: How often? By whom? Were observations recorded? Was person asked about comfort level? Were non-verbal communications noted and recorded? How often was person released from restraint, and allowed to, or assisted to, move about freely? Were effects of restraint recorded such as anxiety, crying, withdrawal, angry frustrated behavior, hitting, swearing, throwing objects, yelling, skin abrasions, pressure marks, leg swelling, bruising, incontinence, dehydration, skin rash, banging, rocking movements, etc.? How much staff time was used monitoring restraint?

6. ONE PERSON AT A TIME—under supervision release person from restraint and place in safe, secure, quiet, comfortable area. Observe and record reactions. Begin by providing ongoing assistance with move-

FIGURE 6-6

PART
ONE
88

ment and balance, interaction with others. Observe and protect against exhaustion and overexertion. After a period of movement, place person in deep comfortable chair. Consider use of safety device in terms of a padded lap belt until person adjusts to freedom of movement. Once safety and functional assessment is completed, provide person with appropriate seating and movement area. Observe and record carefully for at least one week, and work with all staff groups/ shifts. Once a review is completed, move to #7.

7. REMOVE THIS ONE PERSON'S PHYSICAL RESTRAINT(S) FROM THE UNIT OR WARD TO AN AREA OF THE FACILITY WHERE IT CANNOT BE ACCESSED AGAIN . . . EVER!

8. DOCUMENT NEW CARE STRATEGY and communicate to all care staff/families/volunteers. Emphasize that this new strategy is a treatment developed by the team, and is not subject to adaptation by any one staff without consultation and approval of the whole interdisciplinary team. Implement the requirement that any staff using restraint for the person under review must document all alternate strategies tried prior to the use of restraint, and the particular circumstances that warranted the action of re-introducing restraint.

9. FOR EVERY NEW PERSON who walks into the facility or care unit, avoid the use of both chemical and physical restraint, and HELP KEEP THEM WALKING for the duration of the disease.

10. It is recognized that SOME PERSONS WILL BE SO DEBILITATED OR EXCESSIVELY DISABLED that some form of safety device is necessary to assist with posture and comfort. For each of these persons, review their seating and functional requirements. Use an absolute minimum of adaptive equipment or furniture to ensure their comfort and safety. Ensure that they have interesting objects within their reach. Change their positions and location frequently.

11. TRAIN FAMILY CAREGIVERS, VOLUNTEERS, STUDENTS, AND PEO-PLE FROM COMMUNITY ORGANIZATIONS in appropriate ways to assist with indoor and outdoor walking programs and bedside sitting programs.

12. ADAPT BEDROOMS by lowering beds, or using low beds, placing safety mats around the bed, using one safety rail padded with pillows, placing one edge of bed against the wall to increase security. Consider the use of Dutch doors, or gates to limit exhaustion and exposure to the complex and demanding facility when the person with dementia can no longer manage.

PART TWO

ASSESSMENT IN DEMENTIA CARE

7

Assessment: The Missing Link in Dementia Care

He was a man, take him for all in all,
I shall not look upon his like again.
—William Shakespeare

Once the disease process has been identified, the second step of dementia care is the development of the knowledge base about the individual through effective assessment. The effects of dementing illness, such as Alzheimer's disease, are so destructive that it is easy to lose the essential human being in the devastation. As people are robbed of cognition, communication, and rational behavior, they slowly slip from the roles of mother, father, husband, neighbor, and friend into helplessness. And, as we have seen, these diseases have the power to destroy caregivers as well, sentencing them to lives of exhaustion, grief, and poor health.

The focus in dementia care must always be on understanding the specific dysfunction affecting the person with dementia, so that we can design a prosthesis to compensate for the damage that has occurred. We must never forget that large parts of the brain (and the capacities they provide) remain functioning far into the disease process. We cannot stop the relentless progress of Alzheimer's disease; but we can do a great deal to preserve and cherish the parts of the person that are not yet affected by the disease.

This is the hope and challenge of dementia care: How much of the person remains intact in the shambles of his brain? What does the person feel? What can the person do? What would he say to us if he could? In what ways does he need us to help? To answer these questions, we must carry out a careful, multifaceted assessment of each individual.

Elderly people tend to have multiple diagnoses and problems. One diagnosis—one syndrome—rarely accounts for the person's overall behavior. Mental illness will appear with physical symptoms, and physical illness may appear with mental disturbance. To gain accurate information about an elderly person, it is necessary to investigate a variety of domains and assess the whole person.

Quality care begins with a systematic evaluation of the behavior and inner processes of the older person and former social, environmental contexts. Such an evaluation is indispensable to proper treatment. The overall purpose of an assessment is to determine—

- the health status of the elderly person;
- links/tensions among diagnoses, behaviors, and social roles;
- need for services;
- whether care needed is being provided;
- if not, how we can develop a treatment or care plan based on the appraisal of the person's health status—not the system's requirements; and
- how we can best monitor progress.

There are many factors that complicate the assessment process. First, the number and variety of available assessment tools is bewildering and frequently discouraging. Moreover, most of the standard tools for carrying out functional assessments have evolved from rehabilitation practice, rather than having been developed specifically for dealing with dementing illness, and therefore don't provide the information needed for dementia care.

Consequently, adaptation is often necessary. Some organizations actually prefer to construct their own measurement scales, but it must be remembered that such tools have uncertain validity and may produce very subjective findings. Then again, government health agencies may require the use of specific assessment procedures.

Whenever two people meet there are really six present. There is each man as he sees himself, each man as the other person sees him, and each man as he really is.

—WILLIAM JAMES

Sometimes all of these complications, coupled with the sheer volume of work to be accomplished each day, make assessment appear to be a desirable but unobtainable goal. Under pressure, it can seem easier and quicker to just do what feels appropriate, instead of accurately evaluating the person's needs. But it's important to resist the impulse to fix the problem before it has been properly defined!

Assessment: An Overview

Depending on the intent of the evaluator, function can be assessed in several ways. For example, function can be determined—

- at an organ level: how has the disease affected the person's brain?
- at a behavioral level: how has the disease affected the person's ability to perform a certain function or task?
- at a role level: does the disease prevent the person from carrying out social activities or work responsibilities?

These levels of perspectives about function inform treatment or care in interesting ways, depending on what the observer needs from the evaluation. For example—

- A physician or neurologist will be interested in the patient's diagnosis or pathology.
- Care providers, on the other hand, may focus on what the assessment data can tell them about the person's behavior: is the person likely to be violent, at risk, confused?
- Family caregivers will look to the evaluation for information on how well the afflicted person can function in his role as father or spouse.

Each of these perspectives gives rise to different interpretations, and consequently different types of interventions. Functional assessment allows us to bring all three of these perspectives together in determining an effective care strategy.

In dementia care, it is also important to remember that assessment observations must be relatively current, since many diseases of demen-

No assessment measures have value at all, unless the results are communicated to the staff and family caregivers who are actually delivering care.

	ORGAN LEVEL	PERSON LEVEL	SOCIAL LEVEL
	PATHOLOGY	BEHAVIORAL	ROLE
CONDITION	Anatomical, physiological, mental, psychological deficits	Performance deficits within the environment	Environmental & social deficits influenced by values, norms, policies
KEY TERMS	Impairment (organic dysfunction)	Disability (difficulty with tasks)	Handicap (social disadvantage)
ANALYSIS	Diagnostic descriptions (Alzheimer's disease)	Behavioral or performance descriptions ("violent")	Role descriptions ("Dad can't drive anymore")
	PHYSICIAN	CARE PROVIDER	FAMILY

FIGURE 7-1

tia are progressive. In Gentlecare facilities, the goal is to have an initial thorough assessment of each resident, and then carry out re-assessments on a three- or six-month basis.

The cornerstone of good treatment is assessment.

Why Assessment?

If we hope to alter the health status or ameliorate the problems associated with illness in elderly people, there must be a system for gathering baseline information from which to detect change (either positive or negative). Assessment helps us determine—

- if the person needs care;
- exactly what type or degree of care is required;
- whether or not the care needed is being provided; and

- whether the care being given is appropriate in terms of the person's needs, resources available, and quality of care we deliver.

Assessment is the procedure that enables us to secure a comprehensive view of the disease and impairment involved. It identifies the links among diagnoses, behaviors, and social roles, and indicates discrepancies that interfere with a person's ability to function and live. Then we can plan appropriate interventions, mobilize resources, and build an individualized prosthesis for the person. There are five areas that need to be addressed in assessment, each of which is discussed below.

Assessment, observation, and evaluative activities occur at all times and at a variety of levels within the health care organization. All observation is valuable! The information of the neurologist who pinpoints brain pathology, the housekeeper who notices an elderly lady talking to herself in the bathroom mirror, the food service worker who observes that a man ignores food on one side of his plate, the care aide who correctly identifies signs of concurrent depression, the volunteer who discovers that a mute gentleman loves to sing hymns—each tiny piece of information helps solve the puzzle of Alzheimer's disease and other related dementias.

First: Identifying the Specific Disease Process

Dementia is not, in itself, a disease. It is a syndrome of symptoms or group of signs and problems that can be caused by a number of different diseases. Since the path of each disease may be different, it is important to determine which disease is causing the dementia. Therefore, in the first phase of assessment, the following questions are asked:

- What disease is causing the problem?
- Is it acute or chronic?
- Can it be treated?
- Is the damage of a permanent nature?

*Everything that we see
is a shadow cast by that
which we do not see.*

—MARTIN LUTHER KING

- Is it possible that the person's behavior has been caused by physiological factors other than the disease?
- Is it possible that the person's behavior has been caused by depression or another psychiatric illness?

The Depression Factor

As a dementing illness such as Alzheimer's progresses, troubling psychiatric issues can arise, in addition to the problems directly caused by the disease process. Depression is the most common—and most treatable—of all the psychological disorders.

Depression is marked by changes in appetite, sleeping, loss of interest in and enjoyment of life, general fatigue, feelings of worthlessness, and suicidal thoughts or ideas.

GENTLECARE Strategy

Tell the person with dementia repeatedly that he is loved and needed...that the caregiver will never abandon him...that the caregiver understands and will always be there for him.

Clinical depression can closely mimic Alzheimer's disease, and may be referred to as pseudo dementia. On the other hand, depression can occur in combination with dementing illness. It is critical that staff members are familiar with the signs and symptoms of depression, since they are the ones who are in daily contact with elderly people in care; their observations are very important for depression to be effectively diagnosed and treated.

As losses in function occur, grief and depression engulf people afflicted with Alzheimer's disease, especially in the early stages. Care providers who understand the person's behavior, and who can support and reassure them that they will not be abandoned, can be very effective in relieving the person's emotional responses.

Some professionals suggest that as many as three out of four elderly people living in health care institutions may experience clinical depression. More women than men appear to be affected, and women are especially likely to be depressed if there has been a history of mood disorders in the family.

DEPRESSION

For a diagnosis of clinical depression to be reached, at least four of the following symptoms must be present every day for a period of at least two weeks (Diagnostic and Statistical Manual of Mental Disorders, IV):

- loss of interest or pleasure in activities or pastimes;
- sad, blue, hopeless, down-in-the-dumps, irritable;
- mood is prominent and persistent;
- poor appetite/weight loss or increased appetite/weight gain;
- insomnia or hypersomnia;
- psychomotor agitation or retardation of movement;
- loss of energy/fatigue;
- feeling of worthlessness, self-reproach, guilt;
- complaints about ability to think or concentrate;
- indecisiveness; and
- recurrent thoughts of death/suicide.

It is estimated that approximately 30 percent of people with Alzheimer's disease experience a mild depression syndrome expressed by withdrawal, poor sleeping patterns, and poor eating patterns. They may also cry or become anxious. Secondary depression is caused by medication or concurrent illness. An estimated 10 percent of Alzheimer patients experience a major depression, presenting with loss of appetite, disturbed sleep, decreased energy levels, lack of interest in life, and morbid thoughts. Some succeed in committing suicide.

Other major psychiatric symptoms that often present in Alzheimer's disease are paranoid delusions (someone is spying on me, someone has stolen my money); misidentification (mistaking the caregiver for someone else, believing people on television are real); and hallucinatory experiences, both auditory and visual (the person may converse with an imaginary person, see snakes in the bathtub, or imagine burglars are climbing in the window).

I VIVIDLY REMEMBER *the first time I became aware that my father was hallucinating. Usually all of the family slept like logs at night, having kept up with Dad all day. However, one night I heard strange sounds and when I investigated I found my father in an absolute frenzy, moving furniture out onto the lawn. He was sweating and exhausted from his efforts, and the whole place was in chaos.*

When I asked him what was the matter, he looked at me in panic and said, "Can't you see, the house is on fire, there is fire everywhere, we must get everything out!" His absolute terror left me in no doubt that he felt he was surrounded by fire.

LEVELS OF ASSESSMENT

LEVEL 1   General awareness

LEVEL 2   Observational and anecdotal recording

LEVEL 3   Basic assessment of person's ability to perform daily
living activities

LEVEL 4   Assessment instruments to be administered and
interpreted by skilled professionals

LEVEL 5   Specialized dementia rating scales to pinpoint
specific areas of dysfunction administered by skilled
professionals

FIGURE 7-2

Second: Estimating the Degree of Progress of the Disease

Dementing diseases are not static: the conditions change over time, and the needs of a person with dementia change as the illness progresses. Therefore, one must ask—

- How long has the person been afflicted?
- What stage has the disease reached?
- What areas of the brain are affected?

Levels of the Assessment Process

Assessment can and should be carried out in a number of ways, and by all the people who work with the person with dementia. All information is valuable and needs to be considered.

Assessment Level I: General Awarenesss

All family members and health care staff who come in contact with people experiencing a dementing illness need to have a basic understanding of the dementing illnesses and the behaviors they cause. Such an understanding not only helps them to deal with what they observe, but allows them to organize their observations so that they can be used to help all members of the treatment team.

Consequently, Gentlecare uses two sets of formats to help people focus their observations about the functional abilities of a person with dementia: The 7 W's of Functional Assessment and Dementia MPA5CT. The use of these two formats helps to make the observations of many different people accessible to all, and improves communication about care.

7 W'S

The 7 W's of Functional Assessment (*Doing Things*, by Jitka M. Zgola, John Hopkins University Press)asks the following questions: What can the person do? What does the person do? How does he or she do it? Which parts of the task is the person unable to do? Why is he or she unable to do them? Where does he or she perform best? When does he or she perform best?

DEMENTIA MPA5CT

Dementia MPA5CT provides caregivers with an overview of dementia symptoms:

- *Memory*—a person with dementia loses the ability to recall information that has just been made available, and short-term memory progressively declines. However, though the person may require assistance to use long-term memory, all past learning, experience, habits, and knowledge can be used to help compensate for short-term memory deficits.

- *Perception*—people with dementia lose the ability to interpret sensory information. They have problems perceiving directions, distance, and the relationship between external objects and their own bodies. They fail to recognize how one body part relates to another.

- *Agnosia*—people with dementia lose the ability to recognize familiar sensations.

- *Anomia*—dementia destroys the ability to recall the word or phrase that identifies a familiar object.

- *Aphasia*—a person with dementia may experience a deficit or total loss of ability to speak, understand speech, to write, or to read.

- *Apraxia*—dementing illnesses can destroy a person's ability to carry out skilled and purposeful movements—to make the body do what the mind wants it to do.

- *Abulia*—a person with dementia may be unable to hold a thought long enough to complete an action or a communication.

- *Communication*—a person with dementia is afraid of making mistakes, losing a train of thought, and not finding the correct word to express feelings or meaning. On the other hand, conversation may come out as a "word salad," or a jumble of words. Caregivers can assist by supplying words, finishing sentences, and listening carefully for connections and clues. The goal is to help the person retain the ability to talk, as comfortably as possible, for as long as possible.

- *Thought processing*—people with dementia can't process new information, interpret external events, use reason or judgement, or think abstractly. They cannot problem-solve, initiate thinking, or focus and concentrate. Thus, they are extremely vulnerable in new learning situations.

Assessment Level 2: Observational and Anecdotal Recording

Much information about the behavior and performance of people with dementing illness is passed verbally from one staff member to another, or from a family caregiver or volunteer to a staff member. Such information can be very subjective. It is the gossip of health care. It can be distorted. It can be lost, forgotten, or ignored. Team rounds, shift-change briefings, interdisciplinary meetings, informal phone conversations, or mini-briefings while staff work, lend themselves to Level 2 Assessment.

Gentlecare uses two observational strategies to help staff members, families, and volunteers organize their anecdotal information. One is a *Stress Profile* based on the work of Geri Hall, and developed as an assessment tool by Moyra Jones Resources. The second is a technique called *Behavior Mapping*, through which an individual with dementing illness is observed over a 24-hour cycle. Observed behaviors are then divided into categories (sleep, activity, walking, rest, etc.) and developed into a graph or profile of the person's activity level over the entire period. This information, displayed graphically, helps care staff understand the daily life pattern of the people whose lives they manage.

Based on the individual activity profiles, programs can be fit to each person's ability to perform. For example, long periods of inactivity can be broken with meaningful programs. The tendency to bunch all activities into a brief and stressful period should be evaluated and perhaps changed.

STRESS PROFILE

FIGURE 7-3

Assessment Level 3:
Basic Assessment of Ability to Perform
Daily Living Activities

When a person with dementing illness requires assistance with personal care, staff members need specific information on the person's level of dysfunction, as well as his remaining abilities. Staff members are responsible for providing the appropriate amount of help to com-

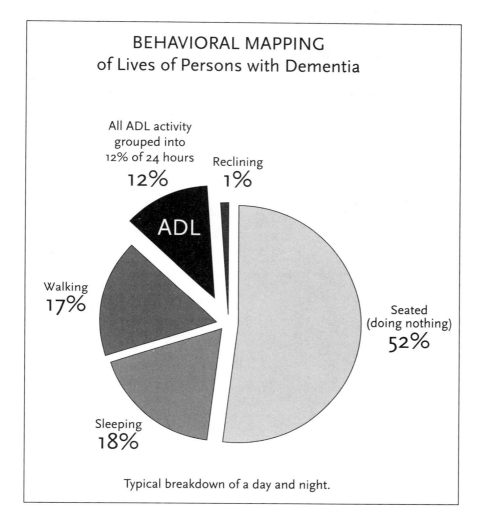

BEHAVIORAL MAPPING
of Lives of Persons with Dementia

All ADL activity grouped into 12% of 24 hours
12%

Reclining
1%

ADL

Walking
17%

Seated (doing nothing)
52%

Sleeping
18%

Typical breakdown of a day and night.

FIGURE 7-4

pensate for the person's deficits. In Gentlecare this is called building the prosthesis. Failure to assess at Level 3 can lead to overhelping, insufficient help, or the wrong kind of help. Any of those approaches result in *iatrogenic* illness (illness caused by treatment or factors other than disease).

There are many formal assessment tools that staff can use to determine the strengths and deficits of people with dementia. The Katz Index of ADL (Activities of Daily Living) is one example.

Therefore, at the hands-on level of care, staff members need specific information about the level of dysfunction as well as remaining areas of ability of the person with dementia.

THE KATZ INDEX OF ADL

INDEX OF INDEPENDENCE IN ACTIVITIES OF DAILY LIVING

The Index of Independence in Activities of Daily Living is based on an evaluation of the functional independence of patients in bathing, dressing, going to toilet, transferring, continence, and feeding. Specific definitions of functional independence and dependence appear below the index.

A Independent in feeding, continence, transferring, going to toilet, dressing, and bathing.

B Independent in all but one of these functions.

C Independent in all but bathing, and one additional function.

D Independent in all but bathing, dressing, and one additional function.

E Independent in all but bathing, dressing, going to toilet, and one additional function.

F Independent in all but bathing, dressing, going to toilet, transferring, and one additional function.

G Dependent in all six functions.

Other Dependent in at least two functions, but not classifiable as C, D, E, or F.

Independence means without supervision, direction, or active personal assistance, except as specifically noted. This is based on actual status and not on ability. A patient who refuses to perform a function is considered as not performing the function, even though he is deemed able.

FIGURE 7-5

Activity	Independent	Dependent
Bathing (sponge, shower, or tub)	Assistance only in bathing a single part (such as back or disabled extremity) or bathes self completely.	Assistance in bathing more than one part of body; assistance in getting in or out of tub or does not bathe self.
Dressing	Gets clothes from closet and drawers; puts on clothes, outer garments, braces; manages fasteners: act of tying shoes is excluded.	Does not dress self or remains partly undressed.
Going to Toilet	Gets to toilet; gets on and off toilet; arranges clothes; cleans organs of excretion (may manage own bedpan used at night only and may or may not be using mechanical support).	Uses bedpan or commode or receives assistance in getting to and using toilet.
Transfer	Moves in and out of bed independently and moves in and out of chair independently (may or may not be using mechanical supports).	Assistance in moving in or out of bed and/or chair; does not perform one or more transfers.
Continence	Urination and defecation entirely self-controlled.	Partial or total incontinence in urination or defecation; partial or total control by enemas, catheters, or regulated use of urinals and/or bedpans.
Feeding	Gets food from plate or its equivalent into mouth (precutting of meat and preparation of food, such as buttering bread, are excluded from evaluation).	Assistance in act of feeding; does not eat at all or parental feeding.

EVALUATION FORM

Name_____ Date of Evaluation_____

For each area of functioning listed below, check description that applies.
The word "assistance" means supervision, direction, or personal assistance.

Bathing—either sponge bath, tub bath, or shower.

☐ Receives no assistance (gets in and out of tub by self if tub is usual means of bathing).

☐ Receives assistance in bathing only one part of the body (such as back or leg).

☐ Receives assistance in bathing more than one part of the body (or not bathed).

Dressing—gets clothes from closets and drawers: including underclothes, outer garments, and using fasteners (including braces if worn).

☐ Gets clothes and gets completely dressed without assistance.

☐ Gets clothes and gets dressed without assistance except for assistance in tying shoes.

☐ Receives assistance in getting clothes or in getting dressed, or stays partly or completely undressed.

Toileting—going to the "toilet room" for bowel and urine elimination; cleaning self after elimination, and arranging clothes.

☐ Goes to "toilet room," cleans self, and arranges clothes without assistance (may use object such as cane, walker, or wheelchair and may manage night bedpan or commode, emptying same in morning).

☐ Receives assistance in going to "toilet room" or in cleansing self or arranging clothes after elimination or in use of night bedpan or commode.

☐ Doesn't go to room termed "toilet" for the elimination process.

Transfer

☐ Moves in and out of bed as well as in and out of chair without assistance (may be using object for support, such as cane or walker).

☐ Moves in or out of bed or chair with assistance.

☐ Doesn't get out of bed.

Continence

☐ Controls urination and bowel movements completely by self.

☐ Has occasional "accidents."

☐ Supervision helps keep urine or bowel control; catheter is used, or is incontinent.

Feeding

☐ Feeds self without assistance.

☐ Feeds self except for getting assistance in cutting meat or buttering bread.

☐ Receives assistance in feeding or is fed partly or completely by using tubes or intravenous fluids.

Assessment Level 4: More Intensive Assessment Instruments

There are also instruments for assessing ADL performance abilities that are more technical, such as the Barthel and the modified Klein-Bell tests. These must be administered and interpreted by skilled professionals who have studied them and had extensive experience in using them to determine and interpret levels of function. The information gathered through these protocols must be interpreted and displayed so that it can be used by all caregivers.

Assessment Level 5: Specialized Dementia Rating Scales

Finally, there are specialized assessment tools that are used specifically to pinpoint problem areas in people with dementia. Three such tools are the Cognitive Performance Test, the Global Deterioration Scale, and the Hierarchical Dementia Scale. They must be administered and interpreted by skilled professionals.

Third: Determining the Person's Resources and Limitations

A functional assessment is the systematic attempt to measure objectively the level at which a person is able to function in a variety of areas. It evaluates the person's integration of mental, physical, socio-cultural, and spiritual states as they interact. A functional assessment of performance answers the following questions:

- Who is this person?
- How much of the person remains intact?
- What work did the person do when healthy?
- What were the person's life accomplishments?
- What does this person feel?
- Who is important to this person?
- What does this person say?
- What would this person say if speech were possible?

More often than not, symptoms of disease will manifest themselves in functional performance (i.e., the person's ability to do things). Even though non-medical interventions will not stop the disease process, they will alleviate a lot of distress for the individual, his family, and caretakers. Thus symptoms are reduced.

—ALIX MCGINITY, OCCUPATIONAL THERAPIST

See the Gentlecare Model for Assessment on page 110.

AN OLD GENTLEMAN *and his wife had returned to the young neurologist's office for a regular checkup. As the doctor entered the office, the gentleman began the visit by saying, "Listen, Sonny: two and two are six, and that's all I want to hear about that!"*

There is no place like home.

Fourth: Reviewing the Health Status of the Primary Caregiver

Because of the powerful bond between the afflicted person and primary caregiver, it is important to have assessment data on the caregiver's ability to manage the burden of care. The Zarit Caregiver Burden Scale is very useful in this regard (see Figure 7.1).

The less competent an individual is, the more the environment accounts for his or her dysfunction.

Fifth: Impact of the Environment

The emotional status, behavior, and performance ability of all people are affected by the environment in which they live—and this is no less true of people with dementia. Consequently, in assessing their functional abilities, we must consider the impact of their living environment. We must ask:

- Is the environment familiar, normal, comfortable?
- Are stimulants in the environment appropriate, excessive, or absent?
- Is the layout confusing?
- Are there wayfinding cues that the person can use?
- Are there invasive systems (alarms, telephones, intercoms, TV) that frighten and confuse the person?

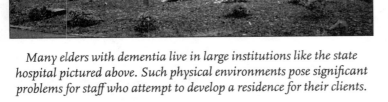

Many elders with dementia live in large institutions like the state hospital pictured above. Such physical environments pose significant problems for staff who attempt to develop a residence for their clients.

CAREGIVER BURDEN SCALE

1–18 MONTHS

Caregiver anxious to provide best care possible for loved one.
Manages the person with dementia. Maintains the house, garden,
and car. Attends to family. "Keeps up appearances." Helps person
with dementia through social situations. Remains optimistic, caring,
supportive. Operates as "Superwoman/Superman." Attends to
personal care. Denies problems.

AT 21 MONTHS

Caregiver begins to take medications, usually for sleep or
headaches. It becomes harder and harder to keep on top of things.
Some help from family is still available.

24–32 MONTHS

Emotional and physical resources are drained. Less and less contact
with people, doctor/dentist/minister/friends. Experience feelings of
powerlessness. Caregiving consumes the whole day and night.
Outside help dwindles away.

AT 32 MONTHS

Stress becomes harder to conceal. Caregiver begins taking
tranquilizers. Begins using medication for musculoskeletal pain.
Sleep is continually disturbed. Caregiver becomes irritable. Less and
less contact with others is made. There is danger of abuse.

BY 38 MONTHS

Caregiver feels unhealthy. Finds it hard to get up in the morning.
Never feels rested. May have hypertension/colitis. Symptoms of
chronic fatigue. Caregiver loses the will to take care of self.
Is unable to manage the household. Rarely socializes with others.
Feels helpless, guilty, a failure.

AFTER 5 YEARS

Chronic state of fatigue. Caregiver is in a state of "unwell-ness." Is
unable to ask for help. Becomes isolated. Is unable to access
resources for information. Burnout is systemic.

FIGURE 7-7

Material adapted from a study at Chicago University College of Nursing.

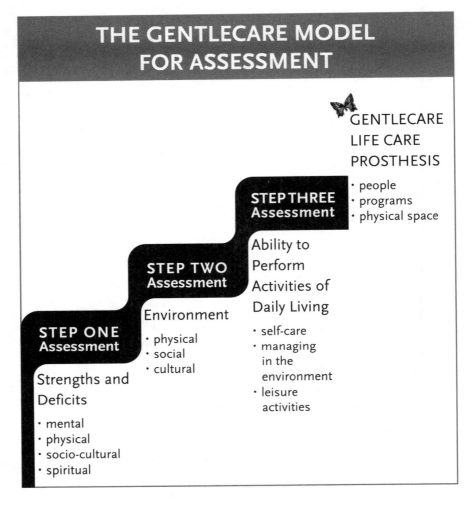

THE GENTLECARE MODEL FOR ASSESSMENT

GENTLECARE
LIFE CARE
PROSTHESIS
· people
· programs
· physical space

STEP THREE
Assessment

Ability to
Perform
Activities of
Daily Living

· self-care
· managing
  in the
  environment
· leisure
  activities

STEP TWO
Assessment

Environment

· physical
· social
· cultural

STEP ONE
Assessment

Strengths and
Deficits

· mental
· physical
· socio-cultural
· spiritual

FIGURE 7-8

- Is there appropriate figure/ground definition?
- Are the colors that are used in the environment easily seen by the person?
- Is there a private comforting space where the person can retreat?
- Does the person have any control of personal space?

The Gentlecare Model for Assessment

Assessment is a complex procedure concerned with every aspect of the client's capacity—mental, physical, social, cultural, and spiritual. As well, it focuses on the match between the person's capacity and ability to live and survive in the environment.

The Gentlecare assessment model demonstrates a way of organizing information gathered at all levels of assessment. The model suggests four steps:

Step 1: deriving information on the person's abilities and limitations;

Step 2: gathering information about the environmental filter through which the person experiences the world;

Step 3: evaluating performance of the person with dementia; and

Step 4: bringing all the information together to design a prosthesis of care.

Step 1: Deriving Information on the Person's Abilities and Limitations

Mental Component

The mental component refers to the total intellectual and emotional response of an individual to the macro-environment. A huge array of complex and interrelating aspects of mental function must be evaluated in this category, among them:

STEP ONE
Assessment

Strengths and Deficits

- mental
- physical
- socio-cultural
- spiritual

Orientation

- Does the person know who he or she is?
- Does he know where he is?
- Does she lose her way?
- Is orientation to time/place/person impaired?

Cognition

Cognitive skills are determined by observing—

- expressive communication
- problem-solving
- ability to follow instructions
- memory/memory processing
- attention to detail

- ability to accept responsibility
- judgement
- reasoning
- ability to abstract
- ability to sequence
- reality orientation
- ability to communicate needs
- ability to do a simple task
- ability to understand and follow directions
- Ability to recall information from minutes before
- Ability to put on clothing in correct order
- Understanding how to transform flour into muffins
- Being centered in the here and now, as opposed to operating in another time frame.

Mood and affect

These two aspects of mental capacity refer to the state of the person's feelings, and the appropriateness of the person's expression of those feelings. For example, a person may be in a state of grief and sadness (mood) due to the death of a loved one. Feelings (affect) may be expressed by withdrawing or being angry. Assessment clarifies both the level and the appropriateness of feelings.

Due to the pathology of Alzheimer's disease as it affects the limbic system, from the very onset of the disease the afflicted person may exhibit rapid shifts in moods, and this can be very alarming for caregivers. Such rapid shifts in moods have given rise to the myth prevalent in dementia care that people afflicted with Alzheimer's disease are unpredictable. On the contrary, behavior can be accurately predicted if the caregiver knows what signs and symptoms to look for:

- Is the person sad or withdrawn from life activity?
- Is the person anxious? Is the degree of anxiety appropriate given the circumstances of the moment?
- How are the feelings being translated into actions?

Behavior

This refers to all actions taken by the person. Assessment strategies measure the appropriateness of the person's action and ability to control behavior.

- Is the person hoarding or stealing?
- Is the person exhibiting behavior that bothers others?
- Destroying the clothing or property of others?
- Lying on someone else's bed?
- Does the person appear suspicious, angry, or intrusive?
- Is the person exhibiting behavior that bothers others?
- Does the person strike out at others?
- Does the person engage in activity that is not socially acceptable, such as undressing in public, masturbating in public, taking out dentures in public, or urinating in public?
- Does behavior appear unpredictable or unexpected?

Perception

Perception refers to a person's awareness of reality and visual/spatial awareness. Damage in the area of perception (parietal lobe damage) may result in hallucinations: the affected person may "hear" imaginary voices, "see" visions, and experience tastes and sensations that don't refer to real conditions.

It is believed that significant numbers of persons with dementia experience terrifying and disturbing hallucinations, but treatment for this psychiatric phenomenon is rarely offered. Frequently, the "crazy" things said or done by elderly people with dementia are a source of amusement or labeling. Neglect or exploitation of such illness is, of course, tantamount to abuse.

Hallucinations are imaginary, sensory feelings.
Delusions are imaginary or distorted thoughts.

- Does the person appear to perceive things correctly?
- Can she tell the difference between someone on TV and a real person?
- Does he recognize himself in a mirror or photograph?
- Does she avoid an area of glare or shine on the floor as though it were a pool of water or a sheet of ice?

- Does he avoid walking on a dark-colored area of the floor as though it were a pit or hole?
- Does she react to patterns on walls or bed covers as though they were moving objects?
- Does he misinterpret noises—the sound of a branch hitting against a window, for instance? Someone entering a room? A public address system?

Thought content

This aspect of mental function refers to—
- clarity of thinking
- appropriateness of thoughts
- organization of thinking patterns
- compulsiveness

Compulsiveness refers to preoccupations, compulsions, rituals, and phobias that may lead to delusional thinking. People so affected may believe others are stealing their things when they have, in fact, misplaced and forgotten them due to memory loss. They may feel that they have been deliberately left out, talked about, or even persecuted. A common persecution delusion is that a person has not been given a meal. Abandoned by memory, the person sees others eating but does not remember having eaten, and feels neglected or wronged. The person cannot respond to reasoning.

It is important to remember that some real event or factual trigger may have led a person to misinterpret information. Caregivers can help by carefully examining the hallucinatory or delusional behavior of the person with dementia. Every effort should be made to remove any identified stimulant and provide appropriate psychiatric treatment. Both lay caregivers and professional care providers need to understand this aspect of dementing illness, because only they can observe and pass on the vital bits of information that permit medical staff to formulate appropriate treatment. Examples of critical information include—
- Does the person evade questions?
- Does his conversation indicate appropriate thinking?

- Does she feel others are out to get her?
- Does one thought follow another logically?

Emotional defence

This refers to the use of denial or projection. From time to time I hear people with dementia labeled as "blamers." When an elderly person with dementia projects responsibility for various actions onto other people, they are using a very common emotional defence! Projection or blaming deflects attention from ourselves to someone else. It relieves us of responsibility and/or negative attention.

- Does the person withdraw from stress, responsibilities, and expectations?
- Does he blame others for his problems?
- Does she try to deflect questions?

IMAGINE THAT YOU *are sitting in a room with your purse or briefcase. You are called away to the phone, and when you return, your possessions are missing. What do you think? What do you say?*

The majority of us healthy, normal folks say something like, "Who stole my purse?!" Think about this the next time you are tempted to call an elderly dementia victim a blamer, or suspicious, or paranoid when, due to memory loss, that person thinks their possessions have been stolen.

Reaction/adaptability

This aspect of mental function refers to a person's ability to live with situations and other people, to adapt to the damage to the brain, and to manage the dysfunction that results from dementia.

This, of course, is the Achilles' heel of the person with dementia. At a time when they are utterly vulnerable, they are required to separate from their familiar support systems and adapt to a living situation that includes a significant number of strangers, sick people, and caregivers. At the same time, they are expected to use excellent wayfinding abilities and participatory skills, and to have the ability to assimilate a vast array of new rules, regulations, and schedules. Deficits in this one aspect of cognition alone would present any one of us with formidable problems. Caregivers need to ask these questions:

- Does the person withdraw?
- Does he follow instruction? Can he?
- Does she follow others' lead?
- Does the person seem frustrated, angry, agitated, or helpless?
- Does he use compensatory behavior to overcome his disabilities, such as walking, talking randomly, clinging to others, asking repeated questions, hiding, going into catastrophic behavior?

Body image

This refers to the part of thought processing that results in our perception of ourselves as old or young, thin or fat, tall or short, and so on.

- Does the person see only one-half of his body?
- Does she recognize herself in a mirror or photograph?
- Does he perceive himself as younger than he is?

> YOU'VE PROBABLY HEARD *the story of the old lady who was shown a current picture of herself.*
> *"Who is that?" she asked.*
> *"It's you."*
> *"No!"*
> *"Yes, it is."*
> *"Well, I sure was a lot older then than I am now!"*

Damage to the memory processing centers (limbic system) and to the time awareness centers (temporal lobe) causes elderly people to lose an accurate sense of the present; they perceive the time period they can remember as the present. As a result, their "here and now" can be in the early 1900s!

Volition

Volition refers to the phenomenon of will—a person's power to control decision-making in life. This may be at once the most precious and the least supported aspect of mental function in elderly people.

Volition is the basis of an individual's urge to explore, to be effective in, and to master the environment. This, in turn, leads to goal achievement, competency, and usefulness. Human beings put volition in practice all their lives—through play, school, work, and involvement in meaningful activities after retirement.

Dr. Gary Kielhofner's work in *Health Through Occupation: Theory and Practice in Occupational Therapy* contributed greatly to our understanding of this neglected aspect of human performance. Flagrant use of the infant/parent model of care, the deteriorating nature of dementing illness, combined with society's penchant for ageism, gives rise to practices that override, ignore, or deprecate the need for elders to control their lives, to whatever extent that is possible.

Volition should receive an especially high priority in dementia care, because it is the motivating system for every other aspect of behavior. It is the part of human mental function that incorporates information from experience and forms our self-perception as a participant in the world.

To determine the level of a person's mental function, the care team needs to ask the following questions:

- What activities appear important to the person?
- What activities would he like to engage in—moving objects, collecting things, turning over furniture, rearranging beds, or sweeping?
- What was the person doing last year or several years ago at this time of year?
- What plans for the future did she have?
- What are the things for which he takes responsibility?
- List the things she wants to do.
- List the things he likes to do.
- Describe how the person spends most of her time.
- Does the person look for encouragement, reminders, or permission from others?

Physical Component

The physical component of assessment refers to a person's ability to move the body freely and purposefully through space—indoors and outdoors, day or night. In addition, physical capability includes the sensory functions of the body.

Range of movement

This aspect of function remains relatively healthy and intact throughout the course of dementia if the person is not restrained or limited by being confined to a wheelchair, geriatric chair, or bed rails, etc.

Care staff attention needs to focus on how range of movement affects function: for instance, does the person have the appropriate range of movement in upper arms and shoulders, hips and ankles to perform necessary activities?

- Can she put on and take off personal clothing?
- Can he brush his own hair?
- Can she raise her arms high enough to reach food on a tray?
- Can he move from chair to bed to standing unassisted or with minimal assistance?
- Can she cleanse herself when toileting?

Strength and muscle tone

This refers to the ability of the individual muscles or groups of muscles to perform functional tasks through the duration of activities: reaching, climbing, feeding oneself, brushing or combing hair, and so on.

Coordination/balance/involuntary movements

- Has the person's balance been affected by immobilization and/or medication?
- Does the person's body exhibit tremors on initiating activity? After sustained activity?

Endurance

- Are activities appropriate to the person's ability, strength, and interest?

- Does the person show signs of fatigue or stress?
- Has catastrophic behavior been evident?
- How long has the person engaged in an activity?
- Have rest breaks been scheduled and implemented?

Sensation

This aspect of physical function refers to abilities and limitations or disturbances in—

- *Touch.*
- *Pain:* Pain is subjective! The belief that older people do not suffer as much pain as younger people has not been validated. Pain is often the precursor of noncompliance with care, and/or resistance.
- *Sensitivity to pressure:* People with dementia often sit up in wheelchairs for 12 hours a day. Wheelchairs provide very poor support for elders.
- *Vision:* People with dementia experience significant real and imaginary distortions in vision.
- *Hearing.*
- *Taste:* Control centers are located both in the sensory cortex and in the tongue.
- *Vibration:* Refers to unceasing movement, to and fro.
- *Proprioception:* Refers to awareness of the position of one's body.
- *Kinesthesis:* Refers to the sensation of movement, and the state of tension in the muscles and joints. People with dementia have a need to move.
- *Stereognosis:* Refers to the ability to determine the shape and weight of an object by touching or lifting it.
- *Appearance:* In terms of physical capacity, this refers to issues such as deformity, swelling, and skin markings.

Paying attention to pain helps prevent it. Offer a cup of tea, a massage, or a warm blanket.

Socio-cultural Component

Social interaction skills

This refers to the ability to interact with others and engage in various social activities, using socially acceptable behaviors.

There is a common myth that people experiencing dementing illness keep their social skills until the end. Not so! Dementia results in language loss, cognitive loss, diminished responsiveness, and inappropriate behavior. Participation, particularly in large social groups, is enormously challenging for anyone experiencing dementing illness. The fact that elderly people with dementia try to react appropriately and get along with strangers speaks more to their decency and spirit than to their social skills. They just try very hard to fit in. When it all becomes too stressful, they may present with catastrophic behaviors. The care team needs to ask these questions:

- Can this person manage a group activity, a mall, or bus trip?
- Can she engage in social intimacy appropriately?
- Does he "fit in" to a group in terms of social behaviors?
- Does she become upset, angry, anxious, or nervous near groups of people or at family gatherings?
- Can she share support systems (staff members, for instance) with other people?

Involvement in community

This refers to the ability and opportunity to continue to carry out social roles and involvement in community activity (church, golf, driving, family gatherings, etc.). The care team needs to ask these questions:

- What has been the person's involvement in the past?
- In what groups, if any, has he been active?
- Are such organizations a potential source of help for her?

I AM REMINDED OF A STORY *of a woman who, over the years, was very involved in the activities of her church. Now, due to dementing illness, her behavior was somewhat disorganized and unpredictable. She missed her contacts with former friends and associates, as well as the feeling of usefulness and contribution to community that church work provided. Her family organized an educational program for members of the church, neighbors, family friends, and home support staff. They came together to learn about dementia and figure out ways that could involve the woman in activities without stressing her.*

> ## DRIVING TIPS
>
> - Solicit your doctor's help.
> - Explain the issue to traffic control officials.
> - "Misplace" the car keys!
> - Make mechanical adjustments so that the car will not start.
> - Sell the car.
> - Move the car to a location out of sight.
> - Explain why the person cannot drive in concrete terms of vision, memory, and way-finding, or injury to others. For example, "Joe, you drove through the red light!" not "You must stop driving."
> - Provide significant support.
> - Arrange for others to offer lots of short car drives.
> - Ensure that the substitute driver offers the afflicted person a map "to help with navigation."
> - **Ensure that the substitute driver has sufficient driving skills to take over the responsibility for driving!**

FIGURE 7-9

Her successful return to church encouraged the congregation to begin looking at how they could help other members of their church who had similar problems.

Participation in family relationships

This refers to the ability to engage in familiar family relationships and to assume responsibility for one's role in the family. One of the many tragedies of Alzheimer's disease is the phenomenon of role reversal, whereby a wife must assume her husband's former tasks and duties, or the mid-life "child" is put in the position of "parenting" the parent. Dementia also compromises the person's ability to be involved in intimate relationships in old familiar ways that are comforting to both partners.

Another common family dilemma is the issue of who drives the car. Dementia destroys the skills necessary for safe driving, but giving up the freedom of control implicit in a driver's license is a terribly difficult step.

One of the most difficult issues in dementia is whether or not to involve the afflicted person in family gatherings or special occasions.

Families don't want to leave people out, and yet they realize how stressful reunions and birthdays can be for someone with dementia. Gentlecare recommends mini-celebrations where the person lives, rather than large parties at home or in commercial settings.

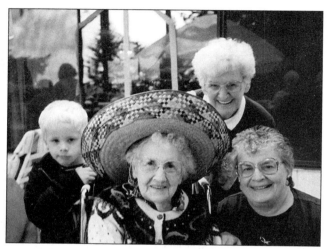

Friends help at Johnson Elder Care, Washington State, USA

Participation in friendships

Assessment strategies center around a person's ability to engage in intimacy, ongoing social interaction, and relationships. Dementing illness causes problems in memory, conversation, and spontaneous behavior. It also causes some people to be more sexually active or expressive than ever before in their lives. People with dementia may forget friends, may act inappropriately, may not talk or respond when others speak to them. They may engage in sexually explicit activity with strangers.

Any one of these behaviors can cause longtime friends to abandon efforts to keep in touch with a person with dementia. Lack of information that would explain the behaviors can cause loss of friends at the very time they are most needed.

I WAS ONCE APPROACHED *by an accountant who told a sad story of a dear friend of his who had developed dementia. He said, "I don't go to see him anymore because he can't talk."*

"But you can still talk to him, can't you?" I protested.

"Of course I can still talk," he retorted. "Are you suggesting I just go and talk to him?"

When I told him that was exactly what his friend needed most, he agreed to try. A few days later he called to say that they had resumed their friendship.

I'm not sure which of the two men was more pleased.

Care teams need to ask these questions:
- Does the person have resources (friends, acquaintances from clubs and organizations, shared hobbies) that could be used for help?
- Do visitors/friends know enough about dementia to be able to visit effectively? It is often helpful to refer them to a support group for specialized training.
- Is the person encouraged to be helpless or dependent by friends/visitors?
- Is sexual interaction appropriate and comforting?
- Does the person's sexual behavior harm anyone?

Spiritual Component

The spiritual aspect of a person refers to a sense of the purpose of life. In dementia care, information about a person's spirituality is usually obtained from close family.

Belief value system

A person's belief system is the set of beliefs or values that have informed his life for as long as he can remember. This value system remains with the person long into the illness. Care teams need to ask these questions:
- Who is this person? What is his religious and cultural background?
- What are her habits and routines over time? Her likes and dislikes? Hobbies? Interests?
- Can or does he exhibit or express a sense of purpose in life?
- What is the source of this person's energy or drive? Is this found in her family role—for instance, as expressed in concern for husband/children/grandchildren? Is it expressed in terms of attachment to a former job or occupation ("I have to get out to feed my cattle"; "I have to go to the office")? Does it come from involvement in church or religious activities? (People with dementia often

assume postures or attitudes appropriate to spiritual places if such feelings are triggered by rituals, ambiance, and activities. Areas designated for worship should remind the person of a church setting.)

STEP TWO
Assessment

Environment

• physical
• social
• cultural

Step 2:
Gathering Information About the Environmental Filter Through Which the Person Experiences the World

The person with dementia does not live in a vacuum: the living environment provided at home, or in a care facility, is a critical factor in the ability of a person at whatever level of function to live with comfort and to perform at maximum capability.

The living environment has three components: the physical, social, and cultural environments. All three must be assessed for their impact on the person's ability to function.

The Physical Environment

The physical environment is the actual physical plant in which the person must live. Together with the social and cultural components of environment, it forms the context within which people live their lives. The following elements of the physical environment are critical to development of the prosthetic of care:

Ambiance

Ambiance is the atmosphere of a person's surroundings, the feeling of a place. It is your experience of living in a space. Ambiance is an important aspect of environment because it often determines a person's comfort level.

For instance, entering an elegant hotel gives an entirely diffferent feeling than entering a down-to-earth hostel. Elderly people with dementia appear to be significantly influenced by the ambiance of a building. Sometimes they talk about "not belonging here," or say, "I shouldn't go in there," or "I can't pay anything," or "The owner mightn't like me to sit there." The care team needs to ask these questions:

- Does the facility resemble any place the person is familiar with?
- Does the place resonate of "home"?
- Does it have a comforting, welcoming feeling?
- Is there some aspect of the environment over which the person can exert some control.

Safety and security

This aspect refers to measures taken to ensure that an elderly person with dementia is protected from danger: not from all risk, but from events or situations that would endanger life. The pathology of dementia diminishes the person's ability to use judgement or reason. Therefore, one of the critical aspects of a dementia care facility or home is a secure perimeter. At the same time, environments need to make the person who lives there feel comfortable and safe. The care team needs to ask these questions:

- Does the facility/home/daycare/hospital have secured perimeters?
- Are security systems designed to be as non-invasive as possible?

Accessibility and mobility

Freedom of movement is the most precious component of care that we can offer someone with dementia. The care team needs to ask these questions:

- Does the building allow clear indoor and outdoor accessibility for both ambulatory persons and those in wheelchairs?
- Does the environment encourage freedom of movement indoors and outdoors, without the need for staff involvement?
- Does the type and condition of flooring encourage mobility?
- Does glare or shine on flooring contribute to a feeling of instability?
- Are there good wayfinding cues in the environment?
- Are access doors "buried" within rooms or clearly accessible?
- Is there somewhere interesting to go?

Function and activity

This aspect of environment refers to the use made of the physical space. The most beautiful space in the world is not helpful if no activity takes place within it. The care team needs to ask these questions:

- Is the space manageable in terms of the person's capability?
- Are the rooms or spaces clearly identifiable one from another, and are their uses very clear?
- Does the environment encourage activity and interaction?
- Are there things to do, interesting opportunities, beautiful objects to touch? Or are they all locked up? Or out of reach?
- Is the noise level tolerable?
- Is there sufficient light and figure/ground definition so that people with dementia can see and distinguish objects?
- Do the activities make sense to the people living there?
- Are activities age-appropriate?

Personal control/comfort/security

In dementia care, physical space can provide the opportunity for individuals to have ownership or control of some place, however small, in their residential area. Areas should be comfortable, convey a sense of peace and security, and be designed to bring people together in small social groups. Built into the environment there should be opportunities to carry on interesting, meaningful activities. Care teams need to ask these questions:

- Does each person have a private place or location over and above their bed?
- Is that private place easily accessible?
- Is the bedroom an obviously personal space for the resident? Are the doors locked or closed during the day? (A locked bedroom means the room does not exist!)
- Are the bedrooms easily identified?
- Does the environment promote social interaction?

I ONCE WORKED *with a client who, instead of going to his bed by the window, used to try to climb into bed with the elderly gentleman whose bed was near the door. No amount of prompting, reminding, footsteps-on-the-floor—not even the fighting that ensued on a regular basis—was enough to change his behavior. On discussing the problem with his wife, we discovered that the bed my client had slept in all his married life was positioned in his room at home exactly as his roommate's bed was in the care facility. When we reorganized the furniture in the room, calm was restored!*

Flexibility

Dementing illness develops over a continuum, and people with dementia have different environmental needs over time. Environmental elements must be designed so they can be changed to meet the needs of residents at many different levels of function. Care teams need to ask these questions:

- Can the environment be changed to meet the person's needs?
- Are choices possible, such as to stay in, go out, go to one's own room, or eat in different locations?
- Are sitting areas designed to encourage participation?
- Can multipurpose areas be converted to different uses, in such a way that they convey their distinct functions? For example, can a room serve as a chapel/dining room/work room/living room— and will it be recognizable in each of those roles?

Social Environment

This is the "relatives and significant others" dimension of the environment; assessment in this area permits a clear description of the afflicted person's interpersonal relationships.

In a care facility, interaction takes place between the person with dementia and family members, staff, other residents, volunteers, and visitors—indeed, with a great number of people. Assessment of the social environment involves evaluation of the pattern of all these relationships. However, in dementia care one truism holds above all others: No one replaces the family! The care team needs to ask these questions:

- Does the person have someone to rely on?

- Does this significant person visit?
- Do members of the family have significant roles on the treatment care team?
- Do they support, or stress, the person with dementia?
- Do family caregivers understand the disease process?
- Do they have sufficient support and education?

Availability of help

It is believed that the average developmental age of a person with dementia at the time of admission to a care facility is between five and seven years of age. Consequently, the provision of appropriate help to people in care is an obvious need. Furthermore, the adequacy of help must be evaluated from the perspective of the person with dementia, not from our perspective as caregivers. The care team needs to ask these questions:

- Does the person with dementia feel supported?
- Is someone available to address his anxiety, fear, frustration, and loneliness? Is this person behind a counter, or right where the person lives?
- Does she live with large groups of people, with no respite for privacy during the whole 24-hour period?

Available companionship

Most people with dementia are separated from life partners, friends, and families. It is not surprising that they often mistake other residents for their spouses or friends. Gentlecare recommends a careful assessment of lack of/need for human companionship as the basis for developing a plan to carefully match people who might bond and feel comfortable together. The care team needs to ask these questions:

- Is someone presently available to meet the needs of the person with dementia?
- Does her spouse need assistance in reaching out to her?
- Do they need a private space or opportunity to be alone together?
- Does the person have visitors?
- Is his room companion appropriate?

- Are roommates carefully selected and monitored? Does monitoring take place when sharing of space is being negotiated?
- Do activities and the environment bring people together naturally?
- Does the person receive mail or gifts?
- Does the person have a special buddy among the other residents?
- Is sexual activity comforting or problematic?
- Is the relationship appropriate?
- Is there any stress, abuse, or anxiety associated with the relationship?
- Is the family comfortable with the relationship?

I REMEMBER DISCUSSING *a man's sexual behavior pattern in a team conference. Staff members were reporting how inappropriate, aggressive, disgusting, and unacceptable this man's behavior was. The team was considering medication, transfer, and restraint, etc.*

One staff member asked whether the man and his wife ever had an opportunity for intimate relations. The team decided to talk with the spouse. Once the spouse and her husband were provided with some appropriate privacy, the man presented the staff with no further sexual behavior problems.

Friends and other support people

People with dementia lose their place in their families and in their communities. Gentlecare works to recreate family and community, to give the person with dementia a sense of belonging, esteem, and security. The care team needs to ask these questions:

No one replaces the family!

- Do people living in the care facility exist within a community?
- Are people encouraged to do things with others?
- Is there a volunteer system in place at the facility?
- Are friends encouraged to visit? Are they trained, supervised, supported?
- Do members of the person's spiritual community visit?
- Do people visit from his community organizations?
- As they provide care, do staff regularly talk about the person's friends and associates?

Staff as support

Many people with dementia simply do not have the support of family or friends. Staff members become very important to those people, forming a surrogate support system. Staff members need to understand that for people with dementia who have no visitors, staff contact is more than merely a pleasant part of the day—it is a lifeline. Since there is currently no medical treatment for Alzheimer's disease, the only effective intervention is individual therapeutic assistance—and staff members provide that therapy!

In dementia care, job descriptions need to clearly state that the supportive clinical role takes precedence over other tasks. While other care tasks are important and necessary, they are not nearly as critical as "being there" for people when they need care. The care team needs to ask these questions:

- Are staff carefully chosen on the basis of their knowledge and skills in working with people suffering from dementia?
- Are staff assigned time to relate to patients with dementia on an "as required" basis?
- Do the policies and procedures of the facility clearly rank personal support over tasks such as bed-making or cleaning?
- Are ways of supporting people discussed in team rounds and interdisciplinary meetings?
- Is a state of anxiety, frustration, anger, or loneliness in a person with dementia viewed as a medical emergency, comparable to pain or hemorrhaging, and understood to require stress-reduction therapy?

The Cultural Environment

The cultural aspect of the environment refers to the system of beliefs, ideals, customs, and values inherent in the structure of the organization, facility, or program. The cultural environment has a powerful effect on the state of well-being of people; it can be a force that permeates and gives meaning to life. It is an element that is vitally important to elderly people, and affects their social conduct. The culture of an organization, therefore, can be a powerful therapeutic tool, especially because customs and habits of well-learned practices are retained long after other abilities are lost.

I REMEMBER AN ELDERLY MAN *who could scarcely walk unassisted, and who was pretty much confined to a wheelchair, which he hated. The wheelchair seemed to represent his worst fears about helplessness and dependency.*

Since there was no physical reason why this gentleman could not walk, we decided to try a strategy: we played recordings of military marches at the time that he was expected to go to the dining room. To our delight, he straightened to his full height and marched smartly off to the dining room. This strategy worked even better when we as staff joined in, and encouraged a small squad to form for the man to lead.

Ability to be interested in others, family, and community

Despite the devastation of dementing illness, most people continue to respond at some level to family issues. In searching for therapeutic modalities to help reach people experiencing dementia, family matters are often a successful tool. Sometimes interest can be extended to the community—for instance, in terms of the person's former involvement in the spiritual community, a service organization, or a community project like a ball team. The assessment process needs to explore these avenues as possible sources of therapy.

Expectations regarding work

The work ethic is alive and well in elderly people experiencing dementia. The loss of a meaningful role as a productive citizen is devastating for them. Work-related activities may therefore be one of the most potent therapeutic measures we can use to help them. Reminiscing about work, or confirming their successes as workers, always elicits interest and, occasionally, joy. Other types of activities such as crafts or games simply do not have the same therapeutic value as work.

It is important to be clear about the use of work as therapy: The work activities organized for elderly people as therapy are separate and different from the work done by staff, even if similar tools and supplies are used. No elderly person with dementia pushing a mop is in competition with a staff member. Employees' jobs are not at risk because work therapy is used.

Expectations of how to behave

Elderly people hold very strong views on how people should behave—both in terms of their own actions, and with respect to the behavior of others. For example, consider the issue of bathing an elderly woman. In that woman's culture, it is probably unthinkable to undress in front of another person, let alone a stranger! To bathe nude in a large room—with a number of strange people coming and going—is beyond belief. To have one or more persons (possibly including a male) assist with the bath is intolerable. Is it any wonder that bathing becomes one of the most difficult tasks to accomplish?

Clothing provides another example of potential culture shock. Elderly people grew up at a time when distinctive dress code was prescribed for specific occasions. One never went certain places without a hat. One wore gloves on such-and-such an occasion. Women never wore pants. Ties and jackets were worn at all times except in the privacy of one's own home, or if engaged in physical labor. Nurses wore starched caps, perhaps with veils. A "lady" never appeared in public without being fully dressed.

Their astonishment over current dress codes can only be imagined! What must they think when they see us work in jeans, gym clothes, or shorts and T-shirts—and perhaps a baseball cap? Do they recognize us in our roles as nurses and therapists? Or do they see us as their children? Could this cultural disparity account for their resistance when we ask them to perform certain tasks? Do they feel uncomfortable, inappropriately dressed, or out of place when they perceive themselves to be in the wrong clothing for events such as dinner or a church service?

Activities requiring participation for acceptance

Elderly people have strong cultural conventions about—
- people doing their share;

- people paying their way in cash;
- people complying with standards, rules, regulations;
- people participating in church or community groups/activities;
- allowing others to go first;
- not taking credit for accomplishments;
- deferring to others;
- being invited to social gatherings; and
- waiting to be asked specifically to participate in any activity.

ONCE UPON A TIME *I came upon an elderly lady sitting alone in her room. Everyone else was participating in a birthday party. When I asked her why she wasn't joining in, she said, "Oh, my dear, someone is having a party but I am not one of the invited guests."*

It is not unusual for elderly people to refuse to attend a church service because they have no money to put in the collection; or to refuse to eat in the dining room because they could not pay the bill. These are deeply embedded attitudes and practices that need to be taken into account during assessment, since they may provide reasons for certain behaviors.

Personal remedies or approaches to sickness and disability

Older people often approach the management of illness in ways very different from the ones we take for granted. Some elderly people have never taken medication; they may view medication as poison and taking it as substance abuse. Some believe that a regular walk, morning and/or evening, keeps them healthy, which sometimes is misconstrued by caregivers as wandering.

Some don't eat if they feel sick, following the old adage, "Feed a cold, starve a fever." Many elderly people have been raised to believe that one simply endures adversity, never complaining, never expecting any intervention. During the assessment process or while evaluating problematic behavior, it is helpful to keep these cultural attitudes and practices in mind. They can often give important clues about the person's reaction.

Spiritual faith

Spirituality has played a major role in the lives of most elderly people in North American society. Traditionally this has been expressed through the rituals of mainstream religious institutions (going to church, respecting religious holidays). Many elders have also had a close association to the earth and its creatures, and have been taught to respect music and books as symbols of our cultural heritage. Some have strong beliefs in luck, fate, or predestination. Whatever the outward manifestations, faith plays an enormously significant role in the lives of many older people.

Assessment procedures should explore this aspect of the environmental filter. It is simply not enough to note, for example, that someone is Jewish. Care staff must examine what Jewishness means for that particular person, and how religious values might be expressed in his present circumstances. The same, of course, would be true for other residents who are Roman Catholic or Buddhist. Whatever the person's source of faith, it is an incredibly powerful avenue for therapy. Spirituality is both intensely individual, and at the same time, of concern to the larger group where there are communal living arrangements.

A word about staff bias as regards spirituality. For professional caregivers, their personal religious beliefs should not matter—nor should it matter if there is disagreement with the religious beliefs of people cared for. The responsibility is to support people in whatever spiritual beliefs give them comfort.

It is not unusual for me to be challenged by staff who hold other religious affiliations (or none at all) when I recommend hymn sings, grace at meals, individual visits by clergy, or a focus on religious holidays. And in one sense, they are right: it is not appropriate, for example, to hold one type of Christian service and insist that all residents of the dementia care unit attend. Nor is it appropriate to decorate communal areas with religious symbols that may conflict with the spiritual perspectives of some of the residents.

However, if we make an appropriate match between a person with dementia and a specific spiritual activity, we can provide that person with great comfort. In dementia care, it seems prudent to assess each individual, consult with family members, and design a program that gives each individual the spiritual comfort and strength needed. Then stand back and watch for miracles!

One woman, for example, who was extremely resistant to being bathed, relaxed and enjoyed her bath when we sang her favorite hymns while the staff member bathed her. The focus on a spiritual practice appeared to change the context sufficiently to reduce her anxiety. Joining in a familiar activity (hymn singing) created a bond between her and the staff member that allowed her to accept help with this intimate routine.

Of course, people with dementia must be protected from overzealous religious proselytizers who might seek to convert them to their own religion. Gentlecare has found that a thorough assessment, consultation with the family, and careful listening to the person's views leads to therapeutic support of the individual's spirituality.

A LAY VOLUNTEER MINISTER *once told me of a woman in a total care hospital who was in utter despair. She was anxious, depressed, and in tears every time the volunteer saw her. When asked what was the matter, she said, "I am so lonely; no one visits. My family is gone and I'm surrounded by strangers."*

The volunteer suggested that the woman had one friend who was always available to her—her God—when she was frightened, when she was alone, in the middle of the night, whenever. If she called, God would be there to comfort her. I remember visiting this woman myself, and being amazed at the comfort she derived from her faith. It certainly surpassed the value of any plan of activity we had thought of in interdisciplinary conferences!

LANGUAGE

Language is often a barrier when spiritual dialogue is attempted, especially when people do not share the same set of beliefs or points of reference. Words like "blessing" or "forgiveness" are laden with various meanings, depending on one's religious background. Professionals can respectfully join a person in their care in using such words, without divulging or imposing their own religious views: "I can see the meaning of this blessing for you." Speaking someone's language often provides deep comfort in ways that are most needed.

—Adapted from Lustbader & Hooyrian,
Taking Care of Aging Family Members
Courtesy of Helen A. Bache

STEP THREE
Assessment

Ability to
Perform
Activities of
Daily Living

· self-care
· managing
  the
  environment
· leisure
  activities

Are the activities we design meaningful for the people performing them? This is the litmus test for all activity programs in dementia care.

Step 3:
Evaluating the Performance of the Person with Dementia

The ability to perform Activities of Daily Living (ADLs) and Instrumental Activities of Daily Living (IADLs) is critical because these are the fundamental activities of independent daily life. ADLs include dressing, toileting, bathing, grooming, and eating. IADLs are more complex tasks that involve equipment, the use of supplies, and interaction with other people. Such activities include travel, meal preparation, cleaning, laundry, shopping, and communication/interactive skills.

Most of us take the performance of both ADLs and IADLs for granted. We are likely to think about the actual process of how we do the activity only if we have a broken arm, or when we try to perform an ADL in a strange location, perhaps on a camping trip in a tent. At those times we may become conscious of the actual sequence of events involved in the activities or the use of equipment, or how we move parts of our body to accomplish the task.

However, when a person begins to lose cognitive function due to a dementing illness, ADL and IADL maneuvers become demanding, exhausting routines that consume large amounts of energy and diminish dignity and control. The simple task of taking off one's socks becomes impossible due to a condition called apraxia: people can't make their bodies carry out the purposeful movements that their minds know are necessary.

The most private activity—going to the toilet—becomes a nightmare: one must try to find the correct spot, attempt to unfasten and remove clothing, figure out where to find toilet paper, and remember to cleanse oneself. The everyday task of phoning a friend becomes a formidable job when one is unable to remember a telephone number or how to dial a telephone.

When we assess ADL skills, we not only evaluate a person's ability to do the activity, but also whether, in the context of daily life, the person actually performs the activity.

It is important to note that the performance of all ADLs is significantly influenced by the environmental filter, with its physical, social, and cultural aspects:

- If the entrance to the bathroom is obscured, the person with dementia cannot carry out the ADL of toileting.
- If a shy person is asked to eat in a large, crowded dining room, the person may refuse to go in, or pass up eating altogether.
- If in a person's culture eating is done with chopsticks—but in the care facility someone provides a knife and fork—the person will not be able to eat.

Performance is the key word in functional assessment. What can the person do? What does the person do?

Performance ability is assessed in three areas: self care, ability to manage the environment, and leisure skills:

- *Self-care activities* (ADLs) are tasks routinely undertaken to maintain health and well-being.
- *Managing the environment* (IADLs) involves those activities or tasks carried out to provide meaning in life and to support oneself, one's family, and society as a whole. Such activity is usually referred to as work. To be meaningful, work should be relevant to the person and life stage. When people are ill with devastating, life-destroying conditions like Alzheimer's disease, productive activity is not just something we provide to keep them busy, to give them something to do. Productive activity becomes a way to give their lives meaning. It is a means of giving them back their lives.
- *Leisure activities* are those components of life that are free from responsibility, work, and self-care. They can take place in the context of social occasions, recreational events, or time with family. On occasion they can be work activities undertaken in a group so that

"Activities" are tasks that engage a person's time and energy.

people can gather and have fun doing a task together. For example, people might go fruit picking, make bread or jam, garden, clean house, or quilt as a group activity.

Leisure activities for people with dementia should be age appropriate and stress free. Leisure activities should not require them to do things they no longer can do, nor require them to interact with large groups of people. Whenever possible, leisure activities should involve family.

THE ADL ASSESSMENT PROCESS

Assistance must be personalized. Gentlecare tips help caregivers to assist with activities of daily living.

Dementing illness causes the afflicted person to depend on the goodwill and kindness of others for help with very personal tasks. And therein lies the challenge for both the afflicted and the helper. There is no more critical component in dementia care than offering just the right degree of assistance! Too little assistance can leave the afflicted person floundering and stressed; too much assistance can be diminishing and frustrating. Like the bear family's porridge, assistance has to be "just right!"

So how do we determine exactly how much help, in what areas, at what time, in what form will give the person with dementia the necessary "leg up" to perform daily living activities , without feeling overburdened by the very help offered?

In Gentlecare, an appropriate ADL prosthesis is constructed on the basis of assessment of the person's dysfunction and remaining capabilities. Unfortunately, cognitively impaired people are often assumed to be unable to do anything—whereas they may be unable to initiate a task, but quite able to carry it out once it is begun. They should be regarded as people who have significant functional dependency, and who therefore require specific help with aspects of their personal care

Questions to be asked in identifying ADL problems—
- Determine the nature of the problem.
- Is it due to memory loss?
- Is it a problem with interpretive skills?
- Is it due to visual or perceptual dysfunction?
- Is it a question of finding the appropriate place to perform the activity?

- Is it a sequencing issue?
- Is it a problem of rush, noise, confusion, or stress?

Determine the frequency of the difficulty—
- Does it occur rarely? Why?
- Does it occur occasionally? In what circumstances?
- Does it occur frequently? Time of day? Who is involved?

Determine how much help is required—
- Does a little help make it possible for the person to do the task?
- Is some help required at the beginning of the activity?
- Does the person need considerable assistance to carry out the task successfully?

Determine what prompts or help work—
Prompts can be verbal: "The bathroom is this way, Mrs. Smith."
Or they can be mimed: the helper acts out the correct procedure and the afflicted person—hopefully—mimics the action. Or the prompt can be physical: the helper can actually move the afflicted person's body through the motion. A staff member can actually carry out the activity or part of it for the person: an arm may be put into the correct armhole of a jacket, for instance. Or assistance can take the form of a combination of these prompts, designed to match the specific deficits and remaining skills of each individual in care. Obviously, no single, standard way of helping will meet the needs of all people. Assistance must be personalized.

In Gentlecare we refer to this sort of information as Gentlecare tips, and these successful ways of helping are posted above each person's bed or in the bathroom where ADL activity takes place.

Tasks must be divided into sequences, so that those parts of the activity the person can do can be separated from the parts of the task that the person can't do, or can accomplish only with a "prompt" or assistance.

For example, if a person stands in front of a sink with a toothbrush and toothpaste at hand, but does not brush the teeth, it can be assumed that the person can't do the task at all; can't initiate the task; or can do only parts of the task. If the helper assumes the first alternative, and does the activity for the person, over time the afflicted person will lose the ability to accomplish any part of the task and will become dependent on others for toothbrushing.

If the helper assumes the second alternative, the person may need only a verbal or physical prompt to initiate the movement, and then will be able to complete the task without assistance. In that case, the person retains both skills and dignity, and the helper saves time by not having to carry out the task.

If the helper finds that the third alternative is the case, it must be carefully decided which parts of the sequence the person can do. Then the helper offers a prosthesis of help by doing the bits of the task that the person finds difficult or impossible. Once again, both parties win.

Here are some ideas for providing effective help with basic self-care activities to cognitively impaired people:

Prepare for the task:
- Have appropriate information.
- Prepare supplies and equipment and space.
- Have a contingency plan.
- Organize other help if needed.
- Allow appropriate time.

Prepare the person:
- Establish visual contact.
- Attract attention by touch.
- Establish your role as a caregiver.
- Explain the task to be accomplished.
- Get agreement to accept your help.

Assist the person through the task
Observe for signs of stress
Introduce stress-reducing strategies:
- information, laughter, rest
- alternate guides
- hot beverage
- finger foods

Celebrate the accomplishment with a reward!

I WAS ONCE ASKED *to work with a woman who, though very compliant in every other way, was very difficult to assist with dressing in the morning.*

When I asked if anyone could help her successfully, one care aide said, "Yes. When I put her stockings and shoes on before she gets out of bed, I have no problem. If I put her bare feet on the floor, she resists all my help from then on."

This procedure may have reflected a lifelong habit; in any event, once this ADL prosthesis was identified and posted as a Gentlecare tip, the staff experienced no further difficulties in helping the woman with ADL.

Step 4:
Bringing All the Information Together to Design a Prosthesis of Care

No assessment measure—no matter how good—has any value at all unless the results are communicated to the staff and the family caregivers who are actually delivering care.

If assessment data is relegated to a medical chart, and not used directly in care planning or delivery, the individual staff or family member will approach the care process in the way felt to be most appropriate. Most often, the result of that approach is overhelping, which leads to helplessness and learned dependency. Alternately, it's possible that caregivers resort to helping too little. That approach forces the person with dementia to undertake tasks that can no longer be performed, which often results in catastrophic behavior.

Information must be communicated to all shifts of staff and to any staff member, volunteer, or family member who might interact with the person with dementing illness. It must be remembered that people exist in a 24-hour continuum; care plans that function only during the day and can be disregarded at other times have no place in dementia care. Consequently, care cannot be planned or delivered effectively on an eight-hour shift basis. Information cannot be held by special inter-

GENTLECARE
LIFECARE
PROSTHESIS

· people
· programs
· physical space

est groups and selectively "leaked" at care conferences or during times of catastrophic behavior.

Assessment data must inform the way dementia care is delivered in every aspect of the person's life for an appropriate prosthesis to be constructed. The importance of "seamless" or "borderless" care across all shifts cannot be overemphasized. The practice of having three different shifts singing from three different songbooks is devastating for people with dementing illness. It also leads to accelerated tension among teams of staff; to competition; and to scapegoating. It results in the waste of creative energy and general loss of focus in delivery of care.

The Gentlecare strategy recommends rotating individual staff members through various shifts for orientation purposes only, to improve awareness of care issues, respect for individuals, and understanding of all aspects of dementia care work.

The need for that sort of awareness, respect, and understanding is illustrated by the following scenario, which is only too typical:

A CARE AIDE REPORTS *that a person is exhibiting "violent" behavior—and medication is often prescribed on the basis of such a report. When the care aide is asked to explain the context of the person's behavior, the response usually is a comment like, "When I approached Mr. B. from the side of his wheelchair, he just lashed out at me!" At this point, some professional will usually explain to the care aide that this behavior probably occurred because Mr. B has lost peripheral vision, which meant that he couldn't see anyone approaching from the side. He was probably frightened or threatened by the sudden appearance of a person in front of him, which produced a predictable defensive response.*

But this information, in effect, has come too late. Functional assessment data, appropriately communicated to all staff, family, and volunteers, would have prevented the event, and avoided the stress of fear for both the man and the care aide.

It is also important to remember that in the development of care plans, the assessment data used must be relatively current, since many diseases of dementia are progressive. A person's condition can change from day to day. The goal of facilities that practice Gentlecare is to have a thorough assessment of every person immediately on acceptance and then to carry out reassessments of all patients on a three-month or six-month basis. A person's ADL status is dynamic. As staff members become more skilled in assessment procedures, evaluation of ADL status can occur more frequently and efficiently.

DEFICITS DUE TO DEMENTIA

	Frontal Lobe Dysfunction	Sensory	Language and Communication	Movement
GENERAL	Problems with reasoning, judgment, personality, and social mores.	May result in agnosia, hallucinations, seizures, delusions.	Results in communication disability, aphasia, anomia.	Results in apraxia.
EATING	Person may take out dentures, eat with hands, "steal" others' food, or make inappropriate noises or actions.	Person may not be able to distinguish food from toxic, distasteful, or other harmful substances.	Person may be unable to express preferences, engage in social conversation, or make wishes known.	Although hungry, person may be unable to pick up eating utensil.
TOILETING	Person may void in public without concern for social considerations.	Person may interpret wastebasket as the toilet, or substitute an object for toilet.	Unable to ask for help or directions.	Due to apraxia, person can't manage zipper or clothing or cleanse self.
BATHING	Person may misinterpret personal care as sexual activity, may perceive technical equipment as dangerous.	Person may not distinguish hot from cold, soap from food, hair washing from drowning.	Person may not understand performance requirements, may not be able to express fears or needs.	Person may not be able to dress or undress, comply physically with instructions, or initiate movement.
DRESSING	Person may undress in public, or may appear in socially unacceptable clothing, or soiled clothing.	Person may wear inappropriate clothing for the climate.	Person may not be able to express choices or wishes regarding clothing.	Person may not be able to manage buttons or zippers or other skills required to put on clothing, or may reverse the order.
GROOMING	Person may take out dentures in public, or perform grooming tasks in public view, or not be aware of body odor or lack of hygiene.	Person may eat toothpaste, or mix up various supplies and equipment, or not be aware of body odor or lack of hygiene.	Person may not be able to ask for assistance, or be able to explain needs or wishes.	Person may not be able to initiate movement for personal care or distinguish toothpaste from toothbrush.

FIGURE 7-10

PART THREE

A NEW APPROACH TO PROGRAMS

8

Powerpoint Programs: Building the Prosthesis

You cannot create memory,
but you can create an experience
that is as powerful as memory.

Programming may be the most misunderstood aspect of dementia care. It is certainly the most neglected. Traditionally the program in gerontological care has referred to the various activities organized by recreation or activities personnel. Incredible offerings of every imaginable leisure and recreational activity are organized to give older people pleasure, exercise, educational, and social opportunities.

However, when people are not engaged in leisure activities there is no emphasis on program. Mealtimes are not considered part of the program; preparation for the day is not part of the program; interactions with care staff are not part of the program; scheduling isn't part of the program, nor is medical care, bath time, or any other activity of daily life. Critical aspects of the person's life care are not considered to be "program." Gentlecare considers any activity the person engages in, from wake-up to sleep, to be part of their program.

The reactions of different people to activity programs can vary tremendously. I recall one elderly man suffering from dementia who, with tears in his eyes, told me, "I feel like a trained monkey." On the other hand, a cognitively alert older man said to me, "If I had known old age would be so much fun I'd have gotten old sooner."

What accounts for these dramatically different reactions to activity programming? I believe the answer lies in an understanding of the pathology surrounding the diseases that afflict older people.

In health care services designed for elderly people, there is a tendency to regard all the people as belonging to a homogeneous group, and gerontological health care services are essentially group focused. Although at the medical level there is acknowledgment of the difference between, for example, someone who has had a heart attack and someone with Alzheimer's disease, at the operational level people with these two medical problems are provided virtually identical care. People dealing with these two distinctly different health care problems may share a room, eat meals in the same dining area, be cared for by the same staff with no specialized training in the effects of either condition, be subjected to the same routines and schedules, and be expected to engage in the same activity programs.

No other area of health care services operates this way! The care offered a teenager with cancer varies dramatically from the services provided to a youth with schizophrenia. An adult having a baby is cared for differently than an adult of the same age experiencing breast cancer. Even within physical health care categories, different types of services are offered by differently qualified staff members.

However, when we offer health care services to elderly people, the focus is on managing large groups of people as equally and routinely as possible. The individual whose needs differ from the norm is frequently considered problematic. And more likely than not, that person is experiencing a disease that inflicts cognitive impairment on its victim.

Different People, Different Needs

Cognitively alert older people who need assistance with accommodation, meals, and management of their physical illnesses are often able to explore new undertakings, learn new skills, make new friends, even travel, as they may never have before in their lives. Many become very skilled in the production of crafts, entering contests and preparing articles for sale at bazaars and in gift shops. It is not unusual for staff and clients in care facilities to spend months preparing for an elaborate fund-raising event. Often the walls in health care facilities are decorated with beautiful crafts, and some older people can make pin money by selling their creations.

Conversely, people experiencing dementing illness need help just to stay alive, to manage the most basic self-care functions, and to cope with the challenges of interacting with others in a strange and frightening environment. People with dementing illness don't fit in. They can't do things. They mess up our carefully crafted schedules and routines. They are untidy. They break things or take them apart, and they eat the plants! They resist being told what to do, and when to do it. They don't act like old people are expected to.

An elderly gentleman who has attained the chronological age of seventy-eight may in fact be able to operate only at the developmental age of seven. Does this affect his ability to participate in general daily routines and programs? You bet it does! The different needs of people in care must inform the type of programs we build to help them through the rest of their lives.

Monthly activity calendar.

Unfortunately, as the epidemic of progressive dementing illness has swept through long-term health care services, very little change has occurred in programming to accommodate differences in functioning. At best, people suffering from dementia have been accommodated on the periphery of programs; at worst, they are made to take part in programs designed for cognitively alert elders, and are expected to perform at levels well beyond their remaining capabilities. Often they are banished, or medicated, due to "unacceptable" behavior. But most often there is no place for them at all in these intensive activities, and they are condemned to sit—doing nothing—for extended periods of time, or to walk aimlessly in empty corridors.

Survey data and experience indicates that 90 percent of all activities/recreational resources are utilized by a minority of the residents (between 10 to 30 percent) in any care facility. These people are cognitively alert, physically disabled elders who are assertive, articulate, and often hold positions of power on resident councils. They have developed a high skill level in some craft or are accustomed to social activities such as card games, bus trips, bingos, happy hours, etc. They are without doubt favorites of the staff, as they are interesting, communicative, and productive people. They also have obvious physical illnesses that can be observed.

On the other hand, 60 to 70 percent of the population in any long-term care facility is made up of people who are no longer capable of productive complex work. They are difficult to communicate with, cannot advocate for themselves, are distractible, messy, disruptive, and capable of becoming very upset, even abusive, when involved in group activities. And all this is particularly exasperating because they don't look sick!

There are many factors that contribute to this unequal situation:

- Health care services for the elderly are group focused. Staffing levels are not set to accommodate individualized interventions.

- Staff employed for recreational/leisure activities are often hired because they excel at some sport or craft. Few have specific current training about dementing illness or are aware of the deficits it causes in elderly people. Consequently, activity programs tend to either challenge elders inappropriately or infantilize them.

- Boards of directors, administrators, families, and members of the public enjoy the decorations, elaborate activity schedules, annual bazaars, and seasonal activities that are part of the recreational program at most care facilities. They like to see residents doing "normal" things, like dances and bingos. Consequently, there is a great deal of external pressure on activities staff to continue to carry out the same type of programs they have organized for years.

- Working with cognitively alert elders is thought to be easier than

Frequently, when we offer health care services to elderly people, the focus is on managing large groups of people as equally and routinely as possible.

trying to involve people afflicted with dementia. There is a bias toward providing programs for high-level functioning people at the expense of those who have more difficulty performing effectively.

- There is a perception that people experiencing dementia can't do anything—so why bother? This perception has led to a generalized practice of tokenism: some activities have been identified as good for people with Alzheimer's disease. These include exercise circles, walking, singing, simple crafts, assisting staff to bake, reality-orientation groups, ball toss, and coloring. In truth, many of these activities are not only inappropriate for people with deficits caused by dementing illnesses, they may indeed be damaging.

- Cognitively alert people who are cared for inappropriately say so! They appear in the administrator's office; they petition the resident council; and they complain to staff in no uncertain terms. On the other hand, cognitively impaired elders, deprived of language and reasoning skills, endure, withdraw, or "act out."

- The nihilistic perception that people experiencing dementia can't do anything leads to the practice of abandoning them to hours of inactivity.

- It is common practice to observe an activity schedule for people with dementia that might include an exercise circle at 10:30–10:45 A.M., a music group from 2:30–3:00 P.M., and possibly early evening volunteer entertainment. With that kind of schedule, a person with dementia may have only an hour or two of activity each 24-hour day.

- Higher-functioning elders with dementia may be included in special event meals, large birthday parties, barbecues, or group outings. They are allowed to participate in such activities as long as they do not cause problems by exhibiting "socially unacceptable" behavior. But such activities are almost always outside the range of things that people with dementia are able to manage.

- Social programs are often offered in special care units for dementia; however, staff who conduct these programs are frequently located in other areas of the health care facility and must travel to the unit to provide services. They usually have a variety of other re-

The different needs of people in gerontology care must inform the type of programs we build to help them through the rest of their lives.

sponsibilities, and are rarely able to attend interdisciplinary team conferences or staff meetings. They often work with only minimal clinical information about the people they are involving in programs, and much of the operational information is anecdotal and subjective. Their work schedules frequently prevent them from participating in educational programs that might increase their knowledge about the effects of dementia. This same problem exists with staff who work in community-based programs.

This may sound like a recipe for disaster—and it is! The practices just described have major consequences:

- People with dementing illness are seriously stressed both by inappropriate challenges, on the one hand, and by lack of meaningful activity on the other. This leads to excessive dysfunction, catastrophic behavior, and escalating costs of care.
- Cognitively alert older people are terribly distressed at having to share activities with people who are dysfunctional.
- Care staff are angry and distressed at the lack of programming for residents with dementia, and at the lack of assistance offered them in "coping" with this large group of people.
- After involvement in integrated events, residents with dementia are often returned to their living quarters in a very distressed state. Frequently, staff members coming on shift are expected to manage people stressed by events that occurred during an earlier shift. For example, people with dementing illness are often involved in a bingo game or a dance that takes place outside the specially prepared dementia-care environment. On their return, they are unable to settle down and sleep, and may wander around during the night. Only too often they are medicated to reduce their anxiety and wandering. As a result, these people may be unable to participate in the following day's activity.
- Staff who are "parachuted" into a special care unit to provide programs often suffer major morale and acceptance problems. They are often not considered unit staff, nor are they seen as part of the treatment team. Other staff sometimes feel that "they get to do the

nice kinds of care," while the tough and "dirty" care is left to the regular staff. Often there is a marked lack of collegial cooperation and support: activity staff members frequently report that their programs are sabotaged by other staff who throw out, lock up, or ban supplies and equipment. The effect of these territorial and professional wars is simply devastating for elderly people who are cognitively impaired. They suffer directly from inappropriate or diminished care—but in truth, everyone suffers. Creativity is lost and the joy of working with this special population vanishes.

It must be emphasized that the problems outlined above are not people problems—they are system problems.

Concepts of Gentlecare Programs

The Gentlecare system has been designed from an entirely different perspective, based on a very different paradigm of care:

- On average, 60 to 70 percent of the people in long-term care facilities suffer from dementing illness. Only 30 to 40 percent of the population in such facilities suffer exclusively from a physical illness or a psychiatric disease. Program resources and their deployment need to reflect this reality.
- Dementia causes specific deficits in functioning, and therefore people with dementia require the use of specialized strategies and approaches that differ from those used for people with other clinical conditions.
- People experiencing dementia deserve to be involved in interesting, meaningful, comfortable, age-appropriate activity throughout their waking hours.
- A Gentlecare program consists of all activities that take place over the 24-hour day. This includes Activities of Daily Living (ADL) and Instrumental Activities of Daily Living (IADL) as well as social and leisure activities.
- All staff, family caregivers, and volunteers have a share of the responsibility for developing and implementing the program. Every-

one who comes in contact with the person with dementia is considered a potential agent for therapy or activity.

- People experiencing dementia and cognitively intact elders should not be grouped together for programs (for the most part).
- Specialized activity/recreational staff have responsibility for developing and supplying the structure (or modalities) from which the entire 24-hour program can evolve. They facilitate programs.
- Environments that stimulate activity must be specially designed and adapted for people with dementia, and be accessible to them at all times.
- The program should be person-driven, not system-driven; programs should flow from the initiatives and rhythms of people instead of being based on routines, schedules, or staffing patterns.
- Activities designed for individuals or tiny group activities involving at most two or three people are most beneficial.
- Large group events are not appropriate for people with dementia, and may be damaging.
- Activities should make use of existing levels of functioning, maximizing the person's strengths and interests. They should be failure-free.

A healthy elderly woman.

In short, to structure a Gentlecare program for people with dementing illness, first we review the assessment information and search for the remnants of the individual behind the disease. We try to identify the power source of that person, and then we build a program based on that source of personal power.

For example, consider the portrait of two elderly women in the following scenarios. In the first case, the woman is at home and well; and in the second, she has Alzheimer's disease and lives in a conventional health care facility.

For the first scenario, imagine an elderly woman you know very well, such as your mother or grandmother, perhaps even yourself. Think about her characteristics, interests, and skills. Think about the accomplishments of her life. What does she think about? What responsibilities does she have? How does she spend her days and nights?

Elders need to be surrounded by their personal memorabilia.

Nothing gives comfort like your very own bed.

What are her first thoughts as she awakens? Perhaps she looks around her as she goes through her morning routine and thinks:

"I love that picture!"

"They sure are great kids."

"I better get moving, today is garbage pick-up."

"Sounds like the dog wants out."

"I think I'll wash those curtains today."

"Better get the kettle on."

"I had such a nice sleep but now I must get moving, washed and dressed."

"It's quite cool so I probably will need a sweater if I'm out in the garden."

"This dress has almost had it, but it's so comfy and I can change before lunch."

"Oh! That tea tastes good."

"Think I'll call Mary before I get too busy."

"Oh! There's the phone. Hi! Mary, I was just about to call you."

"I'd better straighten the bedroom before I get too involved."

"I need to think about something for lunch."

"Susie's dropping in. Maybe we could have some fresh tomato soup."

"Oh, the mail's come! I wonder what's in this parcel. Who could be sending me something?"

"Oh, it's from John! He's the best son anyone ever had. It's a picture of the family. Now where can I hang it? Over there by the window would be nice."

Now imagine this same elderly woman afflicted with Alzheimer's disease sharing a room with another woman in a care facility. What are her feelings when she first awakens? What is she thinking about? What might she want to do?

"Where am I?"

"Who are these other people?"

"Where is Bill?"

"What is it you want me to do?"

"Why are you in the bathroom with me?"

"Please leave me alone."

"I must hurry and get breakfast started."

"What do you mean I don't have to do anything?"

"Bill will be looking for his porridge."

"Bill's dead? That can't be true."

"Let me out of here!"

"This is my house and I've got to get it tidied up and breakfast on."

"Who are you?"

"Where am I?"

"Why is that other woman looking in my closet?"

"No, I don't want help dressing."

"Where's my purse?"

"I have to go home, the dog needs out."

"I have work to do today."

"Leave me alone!"

"Why are you both making me get dressed?"

An elderly woman with Alzheimer's disease.

As you can see, both women have similar impulses on awakening: they think of home, family, favorite possessions. There is a sense of pride of ownership about the space they are in, and a natural instinct to begin working on behalf of others. They share a sense of ritual, pleasure in a morning routine that is pleasing and comforting. The perception of home is pervasive. The woman who is well sees her day unfolding before her and looks forward to work, responsibility, and sharing her life with others. But the woman who has dementia feels she is in an alien space peopled by strangers, and no longer in control of her home,

A typical bedroom in a health care facility.

155 CHAPTER
EIGHT

her possessions, or her personal care. At the same time, she feels that her home, family, and work are in some other place, waiting for her.

These alternate perceptions are at the core of creating the Gentlecare program. If we surround people with dementia with activities or happenings that bear no relationship whatsoever to the place where they are *in their feelings,* then it is very unlikely that they will comply with our requests. And much more alarming is the possibility that they will become sicker and more dysfunctional than the disease process itself makes them (iatrogenic illness).

If the objective is to go into a room and waken, groom, and dress the person for breakfast as quickly as possible, then this can be achieved by one or two staff members focused on the task, and working against the clock. Inevitably, though, there will be side effects for the person with dementia: fear, resistance, belligerence, and ultimately, helplessness.

If, on the other hand, the objective is to make the person comfortable in spite of the disease, then it is necessary to change the focus to one of orientation, support, and empowerment. Prosthetic programming is achieved through—

- creation of a home-like environment;
- effective communication;
- reasonable pacing of activity geared to the individual's rhythm; and
- involvement of the person in the upcoming day's activities.

In a Gentlecare program, people awaken naturally and staff provides information about the day, a nutritional boost, a context for the person to look forward to, and personal affirmation. This intervention is performed slowly and gently as the person awakens.

"Good morning, Mrs. Smith. My name is Mary. I'm here to help you if you need me. It's a lovely day, and you have many things to look forward to. Here's some juice to help you wake-up. At lunch time today, I think your daughter is coming to visit you. That's her picture, isn't it? What a lovely family! How proud you must be!

"I think I smell coffee! Would you like to get freshened up and dressed before you have breakfast? You know, I really enjoy our time together in the morning. You remind me of my mother."

IN THE EARLY MORNING HOURS, *Mrs. Flett experiences nightmares that are uniquely invasive, reaching all the way to her heart's core, and their subject, which she can never recollect afterward, is violent. "It's just the drugs," her doctors tell her, "a common complaint."*

In her much milder daytime dreams she drifts through scenes shabby like old backyards, dusty, with strewn trash in the flowerbeds and under piles of dead shrubbery, past streets where white-faced men and women are watering lawns choked with plantain, dandelions and creeping Charlie, lawns that because of ignorance and insufficient money are doomed never to flourish.

In the pleat of consciousness that falls between sleeping and waking she is capable of marching straight into the machinery of invention. Sketching vivid scenery. Laying out conversations, arguments. Certain phrases, remembered and invented, rattle in her afflicted head, taunting her with their rhythms and abraded meanings.

—Carol Shields,
The Stone Diaries

Perceptions that Shape Programs

The way we approach programming for people with dementia really depends on how we perceive the task, and which paradigms inform our behavior and attitudes. Depending on which map or model we use when we work with people with dementia, life becomes either very difficult for them and for caregivers or relatively comfortable.

If the map we use has as its major direction, its major roadway, the processing of a large number of people through various activities so that cleaning can be done quickly and effectively, and the organization can be tidy and orderly, then our approach to programming will be focused on organization, speed, and cleanliness. Following such a map, we would divide the workload between a night and a day shift staff. Night shift staff would wake, groom, and dress people starting as early as 4:30 A.M. in order to reduce the amount of work of the day shift. This is a system-oriented paradigm.

Perception can be challenged by this visual puzzle:

Do you see a woman?
How old is she?
What does she look like?
What is she wearing?
What are her roles in life?

Did you see a young woman?

Or was she elderly?

When you look at the drawing of the woman in Figure 8.1, were you "right"? In the case of perceptions, there is no right or wrong. Each individual perceives the world in his or her own unique way. It is only in the organization of perceptions with the goal of taking action that we must consider the opinions and needs of others.

FIGURE 8-1

PARADIGM

The word paradigm comes from the Greek. It was originally a scientific term, but is more commonly used today to mean a model, theory, perception, assumption, or frame of reference. In the more general sense, it's the way we "see" the world, in terms of perceiving, understanding, and interpreting it.

—Stephen R. Covey,
7 Habits of Highly Effective People

However, if the objective of our efforts is to provide the best care possible for elderly people who have lost their life bearings due to illness, then our behavior and attitudes must be focused on their reality, needs, and activities that comfort and support them. This is a person-oriented paradigm.

There are some who will say, "Oh, all that's fine and dandy, but how are we going to get the work done?" There will be those who say, "We'll need a lot more staff to do things that way," and there will be many who say, "It can't be done." But the truth is, we can develop and implement a different kind of programming for people with dementia, without increasing care costs.

Is my red your red or is your red my blue?

Each of us has many maps in our head. Some are maps of the way things are. Some are maps of the way we would like things to be. The challenge Gentlecare presents is this: to examine our assumptions about the way things are, and trust ourselves enough to experiment with change. Here is a wonderful story about assumptions:

TWO BATTLESHIPS ASSIGNED *to the training squadron had been at sea on maneuvers in heavy weather for several days. I was serving on the lead battleship and was on watch on the bridge as night fell. The visibility was poor with patchy fog, so the captain remained on the bridge keeping an eye on all activities.*

Shortly after dark, the lookout on the wing of the bridge reported, "Light, bearing on the starboard bow."

"Is it steady or moving astern?" the captain called out.

Lookout replied, "Steady, captain," which meant we were on a dangerous collision course with that ship.

The captain then called to the signalman, "Signal that ship: 'We are on a collision course, advise you change course 20 degrees.'"

Back came a signal, "Advisable for you to change course 20 degrees."

The captain said, "Send: 'I'm a captain, change course 20 degrees.'"

"I'm a seaman second-class," came the reply. "You had better change course 20 degrees."

By that time the captain was furious. He spat out, "Send: 'I'm a battleship. Change course 20 degrees.'"

Back came the flashing light, "I'm a lighthouse."

We changed course.

The Impact of Assumptions on Care Programs

Many assumptions inform the way we practice health care. Some urge us to "medicalize" people with dementia: that is, to deal with "inappropriate" behaviors by giving them drugs. Some say that because of cognitive dysfunction, victims of dementia can't do anything—or perhaps it doesn't matter if they do nothing.

Such assumptions have enormous potential to affect the lives of people struggling with these horrendous diseases. If people assume that disoriented people are children—rather than childlike adults—they will offer them children's coloring books or building blocks as activities, labeled as sensory stimulation. Such activity is referred to as "sensory stim."

They will feed people with dementia in adult high chairs or at feeding tables and use bibs. They will engage in a variety of infantilizing activities, including the use of language that diminishes elderly people.

They will do these things not because they are bad, wrong, or cruel, but rather because of their assumptions about cognitively diminished people: they are children, rather than elders whose abilities are reduced but whose feelings remain intact.

And if they make that assumption, and they are the kind of people who believe that exercise is good for both body and soul, they might have people suffering from dementia play circle games, ball toss, or group exercise. In Gentlecare we do not offer this type of activity for several reasons:

- Ball toss and/or circle games are not age-appropriate activities. Elders do not generally engage in such activity in our society, especially in their living rooms!
- Catching and throwing activities require hand/eye coordination and perceptual ability beyond the scope of people experiencing Alzheimer's disease. Such activity challenges them to perform in ways that are stressful and frightening.
- Circle exercises and games require new learning, the ability to follow directions, and mirroring—skills diminished by dementia.

In Gentlecare, effective physical exercise is achieved through indoor or outdoor walks, dancing, and working—all activities that maximize existing function, use old familiar skills, and reduce stress.

A WOMAN SHARED *a funny story about her father who has dementia. The old gentleman had been encouraged to join in a ball-toss game. He had fumbled the ball the first few times it was thrown to him, and watched in exasperation as it rolled away, eluding his grasp. Finally when he did get a good hold on it, he said, "Oh sh--!" and threw it with all his might across the room.*

Of course, I've become notorious for my views on toss-and-catch activity for people experiencing the effects of dementing illness. This type of activity becomes acceptable to me only if the person is in the early stages of dementia, and is tossing a ball back and forth with a small child!

Some people perceive older people as having old-fashioned hand skills and the desire to do things properly, achieving an end product such as a craft. Based on those perceptions, they might offer people with dementia a craft activity—even though a staff member or volunteer would have to do most of the work, and the activity might have little or no meaning for the elderly person.

In Gentlecare, an activity or program is not something nice, extra, or something to keep people busy. An activity is the essence of the lives of cognitively impaired people. Activity is their life—as it is ours! Therefore, when we design activities for people with dementia, we ask the following questions:

- Who are these people?
- What are we doing to them? For them?
- Does what we are doing make sense to them?
- Does it contribute to a feeling of well-being?
- What impact does the program have on the person?
- Have we designed the best life activities possible, given the circumstances?

In the current health care paradigm, programs for people with dementia are designed to fit needs of busy professionals. Frequently we bring a sense of urgency and task-focus that shapes the lives of people in care, which actually reflects not the reality of their lives, but the pace and pressure of staff. Why, for instance, do elderly people have to get up so early in the morning when they have no responsibilities? Why do they have to eat in large crowds, and finish their meal within 15 minutes when they have nothing urgent to do?

Wake-up
All ADL
Breakfast
Work
Lunch
Work
Dinner
Work
Rest
Recreation
Sleep

FIGURE 8-2

EXAMPLE OF NORMAL LIFE ACTIVITY SCHEDULES

Let us imagine a typical work day for a health care worker on a day shift. Activities of daily living are grouped into a rush at the beginning of the day in order to prepare for work. After a brief break at noon, work resumes. After the dinner hour, either some leisure activity or more work takes place before sleep. The day is governed by four major blocks of time: work, work, recreation/work, and sleep. Grouped around these major foci are our activities of daily living.

EXAMPLE OF A HOLIDAY SCHEDULE

Let us contrast a typical working day with a holiday or day off. Wake-up time is usually much later. We have a cup of coffee, rest, and reflect on the day. Maybe we will do minimal grooming. If we dress at all, it is casually and comfortably. After another rest, we may have a late breakfast, visit with friends, or engage in some sport or exercise. This is followed by a late lunch and more rest and relaxation. Sometime in the late afternoon, we may feel a spurt of energy and bathe, get dressed, tidy up, and prepare and eat dinner. After dinner, we engage in social activities, rest, and recreation until it is time for sleep. Note that our daily self care activities are interspersed throughout the day with rest and leisure time activities. The shape of our leisure day is dramatically different from our work day.

EXAMPLE OF A TYPICAL DAY OF SOMEONE WITH DEMENTIA LIVING IN A FACILITY

Let us now examine a typical day of an elderly person with dementia living in a health care facility. Morning wake-up and activities of daily living occur very early, between 4:30 and 7:00 A.M. The person is helped to get ready for breakfast at 8:00 A.M. and then sits in a dayroom, frequently engaging in null behavior until lunch time. After lunch, some ADLs may occur followed by another period of null behavior. After dinner the person is prepared for sleep. As we can see, the person's day is informed by three major blocks of time: null behavior/null behavior/and sleep. Activities of daily living are clustered in intensive periods around meal time and bracketed by long periods of inactivity.

FIGURE 8-3

Null behavior is characterized by a total lack of activity or stimulation.

FIGURE 8-4

This configuration of activities closely resembles the design of a work day for health care workers, with activities of daily living clustered around large blocks of time. The person with dementia has large blocks of time arranged for them that correspond to health care workers' schedules, but because of disease and circumstances this time is usually spent in meaningless inactivity.

THE GENTLECARE DAILY SCHEDULE

The Gentlecare day has been designed to resemble a holiday or day off in the lives of healthy people. The person with dementia is cared for when they wake-up naturally. Grooming and breakfast follow in a leisurely fashion. Dressing may be deferred until after breakfast and a rest, if the combination of ADLs is too exhausting for the person with dementia.

After a morning rest, Gentlecare activity in the form of walks, talks, and simulated work may take place. The person rests and relaxes before and after lunch. Afternoon Gentlecare activities such as music, family, recreation, walking, or reminiscing take place. The person rests before and after dinner, and then engages in some social activity such as music, dance, visits with family, etc. Preparation for sleep includes orientation, reminiscing, massage, bathing, family tapes, prayers, and music. Natural sleep is encouraged. The pace of the person's day is predicated on his or her ability to perform activities, not on the system's organizational requirements.

FIGURE 8-5

| Sleep |
| Wake-up
Coffee
Grooming
Rest |
| Lunch |
| Activity
Rest |
| Dinner |
| Rest
Socialization
Preparation for Sleep
Nutrition |
| Sleep |

A flexible schedule such as is outlined above produces some significant outcomes:

- Cognitively impaired elders are less confused, belligerent, and frightened.
- As a result, they are able to perform more of their personal care themselves rather than requiring assistance.
- The strain on staff is dramatically reduced and less staff are required to support the affected person.
- The normalized schedule of activity makes it easier for families and volunteers to be part of the person's life.

This photograph illustrates the "empty hand syndrome" of elders with nothing to do.

A Day in the Life of A Person with Dementia

These pictures illustrate the joy of people with dementia when they are involved in meaningful activity.

9

Gentlecare Programming

Today, I was a person.
    —an elderly person

The Gentlecare program is based on a belief that activity is most effective when it is an integral part of the daily living process, rather than an "add-on," or a "take-out," or a program that is "parachuted" into a person's life.

The Gentlecare program focuses on and supports self-care activities, communication, family interaction, intimacy, relaxation and stress reduction, competency, and former life roles. Gentlecare programs avoid challenging people inappropriately, and are designed to support and indeed celebrate their existing strengths and spirit.

Gentlecare practitioners search for the essence of the individual, the residual parts of functional ability, the place of power or motivation within the person. We choose activity that resonates for the client, that interests people, makes them feel comfortable and in control of their lives to the degree that such control is possible.

ONE HOT SUMMER DAY *Michael J, my big basset hound, and I went to visit a Gentlecare facility. As soon as the elderly people saw this funny-looking dog they clustered around. Michael always provides an instant activity program. We slowly moved the dog and the group into the therapeutic garden. The staff slipped in and out of the garden, offering lemonade, encouraging an elderly lady to serve us ice cream cones, sometimes urging one or two to leave with them to "get freshened up," returning moments later with a freshly bathed elderly person. We sang some songs and talked about gardening and children.*

I noticed one gentleman on the periphery of this activity. Once or twice he peered through the window, but did not venture out to join us. I took Mike and went to ask him if he would help me walk the dog. He took the lead, and together we began to walk the perimeter of the garden. He began to talk by giving the dog lots of directions: "Come along!" "Heel, heel!" Michael doesn't pay much attention to people's notions of a walk, so there was a need for the gentleman to explain to me how the dog should have been trained.

Then he told me about a little dog who had been dear to his heart, and we talked a bit about his children.

As we neared the door to the facility, the old man stopped, looked me square in the face and said, "Today I was a person."

Normal Human Development

The model used in Gentlecare to develop effective programming is based on an awareness of normal human development, and a knowledge of how performance skills decline due to dementing illness. Figure 9.1 illustrates the process of acquiring skills through normal development, and losing those exact same skills due to brain cell damage. In normal development, a person moves from a preoccupation with basic survival needs, to participation in a family group, to development of a sense of self through life roles and accomplishments. The final stage of self-actualization (as described by Maslow) is one in which an individual operates through integration of all skills, knowledge, and experiences. He controls his life experiences.

Major catastrophes in life such as the death of a family member, job loss, or illness can cause any person to temporarily drop down this developmental scale to a lower level of preoccupation or performance. In dementing illness, however, the systematic loss of cognitive ability causes the afflicted person to lose control of life events, to become inca-

STAGES OF HUMAN DEVELOPMENT AND SUBSEQUENT DECLINE DUE TO DEMENTIA

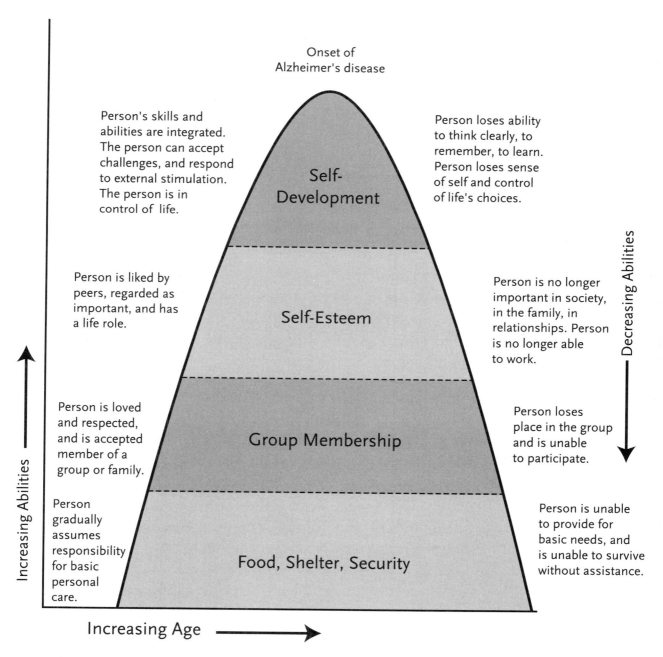

Onset of Alzheimer's disease

Person's skills and abilities are integrated. The person can accept challenges, and respond to external stimulation. The person is in control of life.

Self-Development

Person loses ability to think clearly, to remember, to learn. Person loses sense of self and control of life's choices.

Person is liked by peers, regarded as important, and has a life role.

Self-Esteem

Person is no longer important in society, in the family, in relationships. Person is no longer able to work.

Person is loved and respected, and is accepted member of a group or family.

Group Membership

Person loses place in the group and is unable to participate.

Person gradually assumes responsibility for basic personal care.

Food, Shelter, Security

Person is unable to provide for basic needs, and is unable to survive without assistance.

Increasing Abilities

Decreasing Abilities

Increasing Age

FIGURE 9-1

pable of maintaining his life role or work situation, to be unable to fulfill family roles or responsibilities—and eventually to lose even the ability to care for basic personal needs. This decline reflects in reverse the acquisition of skills in a normal or healthy person.

The Gentlecare model of activity programming has as its goal to design and put in place an individual prosthesis of care that can support and assist the person to move up the developmental scale if possible, or to retain a place on the developmental scale for as long as possible.

GENTLECARE Practice Tip

Give the person with dementia an energizing drink before beginning any activity of daily living.

In Gentlecare we use a system called POWERPOINT PROGRAMS to design programs for people experiencing dementia. Using accurate assessment information, individualized daily care programs are based on the highest point of competence or power of the individual. The process first identifies the current maximum functioning ability of the person—his or her personal place of power. Then the person's current deficit or lowest point of power is calculated. The area of deficiency is the part that must be compensated for by the prosthesis, which is the work of the caregiver.

In standard care of the elderly, activities occur episodically during the day, and different kinds of activities are dealt with differently. For instance, the person with Alzheimer's disease is assisted with activities of daily living or the activity is done to them. As a rule, these activities take place at specific times and within specific time frames. However, other necessary activities such as planned rest or time out occur only randomly and are often confused with times when nothing is happening in the person's life. Planned rest energizes people. Inactivity destroys people.

In current practice, many of the essential activities of life—movement, family, social intimacy, and communication—are sometimes

POWERPOINT PROGRAMS

CORE ACTIVITIES	NECESSARY ACTIVITIES	ESSENTIAL ACTIVITIES	MEANINGFUL ACTIVITIES
The five activities of daily living	Activities necessary for human health	Activities essential for human interaction	Special undertakings
Toileting Grooming Bathing Dressing Eating	Natural sleep Rest/Relaxation Time out/Privacy	Communication Movement Intimacy/Touch Family/Social	Work Play Recreation

FIGURE 9-2

DETERMINING THE PROSTHESIS

The Gentlecare Prosthesis of Care, comprised of three elements—People, Programs, and Physical Space—is designed to match or compensate for the person's deficit. The person is not overhelped or underhelped.

If the prosthesis is excessive, then the person will lose ability in direct proportion to the excess help.

If total assistance is offered in order to make the task go more quickly the person will lose total functioning. This is referred to as iatrogenic illness (illness due to factors other than disease) or dysfunction.

Note marked increase in workload as inappropriate care is offered and client becomes helpless.

I can, therefore I am.

—SIMONE WEIL

FIGURE 9-3

specifically scheduled (for instance, as an exercise group, or reminiscing group). Family visits are modeled on hospital visits, rather than being viewed as a critical part of the person's care plan and a normal life activity.

Furthermore, standard care services tend to define other *meaningful activities* of life exclusively as those that utilize higher developmental skills. By definition, these are usually considered to be out of reach of people afflicted with dementia, who are rarely consulted on the subject or allowed control over their life activities. Standard care rarely sees activities such as movement, communication, family, or social interaction as principal therapies. In fact, such activities are seldom even charted.

Conversely, the Gentlecare Powerpoint Program regards all of these activities as critical for maintaining the optimum functioning level of the person experiencing dementia. All these activities are woven into a complex supporting fabric designed to give people with dementia the highest possible quality of life.

In Gentlecare, recognition is given to the level of energy that individuals require in order to accomplish ADLs. With proper support and prompting, many people can perform ADLs for themselves, rather than be dependent on someone else to do it for them or to them. Some ADLs such as eating and bathing can be the source of much pleasure and relaxation, if appropriately organized. Therefore the Gentlecare program emphasizes these activities, according them lots of time and thus maximizing their therapeutic value. Such activities become the central focus of the day for people with dementia. All staff work to make residents as comfortable, satisfied, and independent as possible.

It is often assumed that those cognitively impaired people who have difficulty performing ADLs are unable to do anything for themselves. On the contrary: such people should be regarded as having significant functional dependency, and needing help with specific aspects of their personal care. Care routines that do not acknowledge existing and residual functioning levels or assess deficits, that are rushed or understaffed, contribute significantly to excessive disability.

GENTLECARE MODEL
FOR PLANNING ACTIVITIES
FOR PERSONS WITH DEMENTIA

Ascending and Reinforcing Spiral of Daily Performance

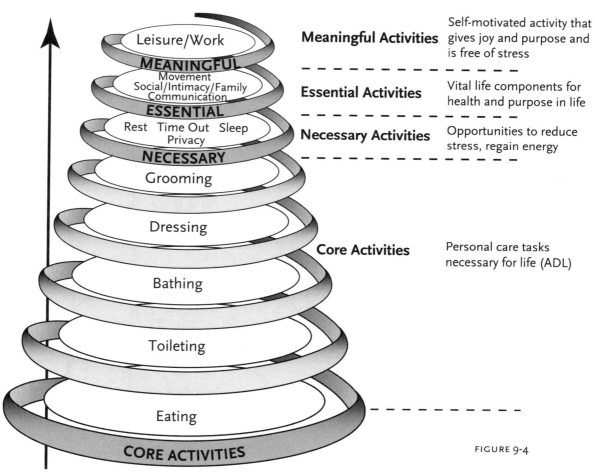

Meaningful Activities — Self-motivated activity that gives joy and purpose and is free of stress

Essential Activities — Vital life components for health and purpose in life

Necessary Activities — Opportunities to reduce stress, regain energy

Core Activities — Personal care tasks necessary for life (ADL)

Leisure/Work

MEANINGFUL

Movement
Social/Intimacy/Family
Communication

ESSENTIAL

Rest   Time Out   Sleep
Privacy

NECESSARY

Grooming

Dressing

Bathing

Toileting

Eating

CORE ACTIVITIES

FIGURE 9-4

Gentlecare aims to build on success in ascending levels of activities
so each person is able to reach the maximum level of meaningful activity.

The Gentlecare Model for Organizing Activity

Core activities are the constellation of activities related to Maslow's first building block of development: the need for food, shelter, security, and basic personal care. In health care, these activities are referred to as Activities of Daily Living (ADLs). However, *core activities refer to the five ADLs as they are combined and integrated into a person's daily life* to enhance the person's quality of life.

For example, grooming is an ADL but in the larger sense, helping an elderly person achieve a pleasant feeling and appearance because a spouse is coming for lunch puts grooming in context, and provides the reason for carrying out the ADL in the first place. If a similar context is provided for bathing or dressing, the ADLs combine to form the core of the person's day—they provide his reason for living.

So although core activities in fact consist of ADL activities, when viewed together they form the basic context of daily living.

Necessary activities, on the other hand, are activities that all people must carry out to prepare for or provide the energy for carrying out other life activities. For the most part, people attend to necessary activities (rest, sleep, relaxation, time out, privacy) without giving them much thought. However, people with dementia must either be helped with these activities, or have them arranged for them. Health care providers must realize that these activities are absolutely necessary to prevent people with dementia from becoming overloaded, overstressed, and challenged beyond their functional abilities. Necessary activities also help give people with dementia the energy to enjoy life.

Essential activities are distinct from necessary activities—and people often ask me what the difference between the two actually is. Many people with dementia manage with only the first two activity levels: core activities and necessary activities. In Gentlecare, however, people with dementia are offered more than just ADLs and a bed to sleep in. Essential activities are the things that you and I do that connect us with other people; that allow us the joy of freedom and movement; and that offer us the pleasure of communication, whether verbal or non-verbal. These activities are superimposed on core and necessary activities to give completeness to the lives of elderly people with dementia.

Excessive disability may be defined as a reversible deficit that is more disabling than the primary disability.

—DAWSON, KLINE, WIANKO, WELLS, *GERIATRIC NURSING*

Meaningful activities refers to the highest level of development in Maslow's developmental scale. These activities are special undertakings that require integration of all our cognitive, social, and functional skills. Achieving this level of development is very difficult for people with dementia. The Gentlecare program helps afflicted people achieve the highest possible level that they can. As people reach each developmental level, their success keeps them with the next new challenge. The ascending and reinforcing synergy of Powerpoint Programs raises people with dementia to their highest level of achievment and the highest quality of life possible.

Core Activities

Toileting

When assistance is needed for this most personal of all activities, there are problems for everyone—devastating the person requiring care, embarrassing family caregivers, and exhausting professional caregivers. The following suggestions, gathered from the personal experience of caregivers, may assist you with this difficult task. Remember to always apply the Gentlecare formula (the person/the pathology/the deficit/the prosthesis of care) to help you find creative solutions!

FIGURE 9-5

Organize the physical environment:
• Clear the clutter from the bathroom.
• Contrast the color of the toilet fixture with that of the floor and wall.
• Place the toilet paper in plain view by putting it on a small stool in front of the person.
• Make sure the door to the toilet is clearly differentiated from all other doors; try decorating the door with a large graphic of a toilet, painting the door a special color, or putting a small canopy over the door.
• Maintain good lighting in toilets 24 hours a day.

Plot the person's individual toileting routine:
• Consult with the person's family.
• Organize the care plan so the person is discreetly reminded, just prior to their regular elimination times, to visit a toilet.

- Support and reward successful toileting!
- Minimize reactions to problematic toileting or accidents.

Discover appropriate language to describe toileting activity:
- Consult with the person's family.
- Make sure everyone is informed of the correct language to be used, and everyone uses it.
- Do not infantilize this activity through the use of language such as "diapers," "pee-pee," or "potty time"; refer to diapers as protective undergarments.

Offer appropriate assistance:
- Offer only the help required to accomplish the task.
- Practice being quiet and invisible.
- Try to place yourself to the side and behind the person's range of vision.
- To keep a person from popping up and down, try placing your hand lightly on the person's shoulder.
- DO NOT USE RESTRAINTS.
- Some facilities place a waist-high privacy screen in front of the person on the toilet.
- Try placing liners on the outside of underwear initially until the person becomes accustomed to the use of protective under-garments.
- Reassure, reassure, reassure!

Prepare caregivers (including families) for this task:
- Conduct regular in-service.
- Provide magazines for the use of those assisting in bathrooms because toileting takes time.
- Unless a person's skin condition is severely compromised, do not wake a person for toileting during the night.
- If a person needs to use the toilet at night, make sure light levels in both bedroom and bathroom are adequate and even.
- Wear mid-range colors, and make sure the person understands who you are and what you are doing.

Avoid the need for enemas or suppositories by providing good nutrition:

- If enemas are required, work in care teams: one member of the team supports, explains, and distracts while the other carries out the procedure.
- Proceed gently and slowly. Do not push through distress or fear around toileting. Try to talk the person through the procedure.
- Observe for pain and/or physical dysfunction.

GROOMING

Refers to mouth, teeth (dentures), eye, ear, hair, skin, and nose care as well as the application of cosmetics. These aspects of personal care are all too frequently neglected, avoided or not attended to altogether.

WHEN I VISITED *my own father in hospital years and years ago, my routine was as follows: I would first embrace him; then I would wash his face and eyes, brush his hair, give him his dentures out of the top drawer of his night stand, put his collar out over his sweater, wash his hands, clean his nails, put his gold ring on—and then stand back and say, "Hi, Dad!"*

Grooming: Mouth Care

I have no magic formula to offer with respect to mouth care. It's the toughest kind of care to give. I only know it must be carried out three or five times a day if we want the person to feel good.

Ask the family carer for advice. Members of the family have often worked out effective routines or tricks for providing mouth care.

I AM ALWAYS ASKING *caregivers for tips on managing mouth care: "How do you get their dentures out? Do you have any ideas about this that work?" One care aide told me she had a foolproof strategy. She said, "I just show them what I want them to do by pulling out my own denture . . . and they always do what I do!"*

In helping the person with dementia to remove dentures, place the person's hand between yours and the denture. In other words, assist the person to take dentures out and put them in. Mime the activity. Describe what it is you want done, slowly and clearly, over and over again. Use the toothbrush and toothpaste to stimulate visual awareness of the activity you want carried out.

I ONCE WORKED *in a hospital where residents' dentures were passed out before each meal and retrieved at the end of the meal. Between meals, dentures were stored in little individual boxes at the nursing station. But dentures are meant to replace natural teeth. They are needed in the mouth for many reasons—talking, eating, and looking your best. A person in care should have teeth in the mouth during all waking hours.*

GENTLECARE Practice Tip

Make sure each person has a "comfort bag" or satchel or briefcase. That's usually where they will put their dentures. Except for my father. He kept his in the toe of his shoe!

Ensure that dentures are identified (labeled). Dentures often fit poorly, and when they irritate the mouth, people with dementia will sometimes take them out and hide them, or throw them away.

Sometimes people will clean their own mouth and tongue if given a clean wet cloth. Remember that the tissue around the mouth (and eyes) is very fragile!

Practice distraction while you do mouth care. Reminiscing and news of family are good distractions. Or give the person something beautiful or interesting to hold in their hands.

Dentures should fit properly! If they do not, and it proves impossible to have them fixed, the person may in fact be more comfortable without them. However, it's best to keep dentures in working order as long as possible.

Skin care

Elderly people often have dry skin, and medications, hot temperatures, and dehydration are some of the factors that contribute to the condition. Massaging hands, face, feet, and legs with lotion is a lovely, relaxing technique for making a person feel marvelous! (Family members and volunteers can often contribute to this type of activity.)

Remember to wash elderly people's hands frequently during the day. This is especially important before and after meals. Gentlecare recommends the use of hot towels, which are distributed before each meal. (Again, this is a good family and/or volunteer activity.)

Hair care

Clean hair, well cut and cared for, makes people look and feel like themselves at their best. Families should be involved in discussions about finding the most attractive, simplest-to-care-for hairstyle; however, old styles and patterns of caring for hair must always be respected. Long hair should not be cut, nor beards or mustaches shaved off, unless there is an extremely compelling reason for doing so, and family members have been consulted.

Touch is ten times more powerful than visual or auditory stimulus, whether from a friendly human, or a favorite dog.

Beauticians should be included in all dementia educational opportunities, and be given relevant clinical information about the people they serve. Brushing hair and massaging scalp is an effective way to relax the person with dementia.

I WAS WORKING *on a dementia care unit one day brushing out an elderly lady's very long, thick hair. We had tied it up in a ponytail, and I was working out a big tangle of hair near her waist. Suddenly a staff member said, "I know how to fix that!" and took some scissors and cut off the ponytail at the point of the rubber band. With a snap of the scissors, the woman's appearance and autonomy were violated in a way the dementing illness had never been able to do.*

People should wear shower caps while bathing or using the shower, and water should never be poured over the person's head. Be considerate: do not wash a woman's hair if it has been recently styled or set. Try to schedule hair-washing so that it coordinates with visits to the beauty parlor.

ONE OF THE MOST DEVASTATING *events in my life as a family caregiver occurred when I visited my father one day and discovered that his hair—which was distinctively long and luxurious—had all been cut off. Only tiny wisps of hair remained among the bald patches. He was unrecognizable!*

I was told that this short "haircut" lasted longer, and eliminated the "problem" of regular haircuts. Years and years later the image of my father, looking like an inmate of a concentration camp, remains in my memory because someone thought it didn't matter what kind of haircut one gave an old man with dementia.

THE USE OF COSMETICS

The application of cosmetics should be done gently, discreetly, and individually, respecting old patterns of practice. Family carers can often provide advice or pictures that can help in this respect.

JEWELRY

Jewelry is a great conversation starter. Like the Queen, many elderly women would not dream of being seen in public without their three strands of pearls! Ask family members to replace valuable pieces of jewelry with inexpensive jewelry that is similar in appearance so that that people with dementia can enjoy the jewelry they have worn all their lives. Costume jewelry also makes a wonderful small gift that can be mailed to the person in a facility. Remember, old men enjoy jewelry too!

ONCE WHEN AN ASSISTANT *of mine asked if he could take a picture of an elderly woman and her husband, she readily agreed but asked if he would wait outside for a moment. I thought she was going to put in her dentures, do her hair, or apply some lipstick. Instead she rum-*

maged around in her top drawer until she found just the right necklace, and then she was ready to be photographed.

Dressing

Clothing is necessary for warmth and comfort, social conformity, and expressing individuality. "Clothes make the man," so the old saying goes, and it is unfortunately true that our society judges people by what they wear. We dress up for company. We buy new clothes for important interviews or social events. Kids wear certain styles to be accepted by their preferred group of friends.

Most elderly people who experience dementia belong to a generation that practiced very strict dress codes. Women wore hats, wore their skirts a prescribed length, and did not wear slacks. Men wore shirts, ties, and jackets at all times.

So what happens to their social mores when dementia strikes? Dressing is a very complex activity requiring manipulation of a variety of articles and materials. Satisfactory dressing requires sequencing: getting underclothes on first, not last. It requires color matching, being aware of right and left, top and bottom, and having an accurate sense of body image. It requires the use of judgement in choosing clothing suitable for hot or cold weather and for indoor or outdoor wear. Socks, shoes, and gloves are worn in pairs, hats must suit the season—the list of choices is endless. So how do we help our family members and clients dress appropriately and still be as independent as possible?

I ONCE LISTENED *to a husband rant on and on about his wife's "stupidity" in not matching the colors of her shoes each morning. He said, "Every time I look at her she's walking around in one brown shoe and one black shoe! Surely to goodness she can see the difference!"*

We talked about what dementia does to one's ability to differentiate colors, and there was a long silence as he thought about the effects of this awful illness. At last he said, "You don't think it's her fault, do you?" And I said, "No, I don't." He said, "You think it's up to me," and I said, "Yes." There was another thoughtful pause, and then he said, "Well, I could just put out a pair of brown shoes, or a pair of black shoes for her, couldn't I? That should make it easier." And I agreed.

Dementia is a continuum of declining functions. It's possible—with gentle assistance—for people to wear regular clothing until they are at the stage of moderate dementia (Late Stage 4 or 5 on the Reisberg Scale). To be able to provide the kind of help that will allow this to happen, however, the caregiver must learn how the disease affects functioning, as in the case of the husband who wanted his wife to wear matching shoes. Later on, as the skill level of a person with dementia declines, it becomes necessary to modify clothing so that independence can be maintained for as long as possible. Here are some of the modifications that help extend independence:

- Choose clothing with wide necklines and wide, deep armholes.
- Eliminate fasteners wherever possible.
- Consider using sports clothing, even though the person may never have worn such clothing before. Gym suits are warm and comfortable, easy to wash, and easy to get on and off. It is also possible to layer sports clothes to accommodate the wild swings in temperature that dementia causes. Discuss these advantages with family members who may not understand why clothing changes are necessary.
- Consider using gym suits instead of pajamas at night. They are warm around the shoulders and lower back, and easy to change.
- We recommend the use of little "huggable" jackets for women. These jackets cover the shoulders and arms, and have knitted cuffs at the wrists that keep the jacket in place. One of the reasons people with dementia wander out of their rooms at night is that they feel cold; they may not think to pull up blankets around their shoulders.
- Some family members prefer to have their female relatives wear dresses. Where that is the case, Gentlecare recommends using long robes with Velcro closings in the back, for reasons of both comfort and ease in dressing. Robes also have the advantage of covering knees and legs, especially if the person is in a wheelchair

or has a habit of pulling up clothing. And robes make elderly women feel special and dressed up.

- Men like to wear vests, and baggy sweaters with deep pockets to put their treasures in. They also often enjoy scarves and hats, worn indoors too.
- If the person frequently undresses in public, consider using a jumpsuit (one-piece suit of clothing) with fasteners either at the front or at the back. Jumpsuits present real challenges during toileting, however.
- Eliminate belts, buttons, linings, or any clothing construction that impedes easy dressing and undressing.
- For a slim woman, it is sometimes possible to substitute a warm undervest for a bra.
- Stretchy leggings are easier to put on than nylons or pantyhose, and are warm and comfortable. Leg warmers can be substituted for nylons and pantyhose, and are easier to put on. Above-the-knee nylons are also easier to manage than pantyhose.
- Light weight leggings make excellent leg covers under skirts or dresses, or on their own.
- Every person who is up and about should wear shoes. Consider using sport shoes or walking shoes for footwear, rather than dress shoes. They are more stable, more comfortable, and easier to get on and off.
- Once you find a suitable kind of footwear, buy two pairs of the same shoe—it will save searching for a match.
- Beware of gym shoes with deep soles and wide rims, as they will cause an older person to stumble or trip. There are many walking shoes with narrow, neat soles.
- Do not use socks with cuffs that are elasticized or have tight ribbing; we prefer socks that fold down into a cuff. Also avoid socks with seams or ribbing on the underside. Buy one size of same-color socks, and lots of them. Socks are expendable!
- And to keep everyone happy make sure clothes are made of easily washable, non-wrinkle fabrics, and give the person in care as much choice as possible in selecting colors and accessories.

I WAS ONCE ASKED by family caregivers to act on their behalf in presenting a problem to the facility administration. What was the problem? They felt that staff was stealing their family members' socks. I assured them I thought it unlikely that any staff member would covet old, shrunken, mismatched socks, and reminded them of how difficult it is to keep socks organized in the hospital laundry. I suggested they try to solve the problem. So they formed a sock committee!

They pooled all their resources and purchased dozens of pairs of one-size, one-color, non-shrink socks. Members of the committee then placed three pairs of socks in each resident's drawer. They removed and organized all existing socks. Of course, everyone was enchanted and the committee received much praise for its problem-solving approach. I heard later that the family caregivers at that facility also formed an underwear committee!

When assisting with dressing identify each item of clothing for the person you are helping, not only by name, but by function: "Let's put your slacks on over your legs so you'll be nice and warm." Offer one item at a time. If you are unable to supervise the whole dressing procedure, lay clothing out in the sequence to be put on. Undo fasteners, and open up the clothing for the person who's dressing. People with dementia may have problems when trying to distinguish top clothing from bottom clothing, often mistaking an arm for a trouser leg.

If the person errs in putting clothes on in the correct sequence, attempt to assist the person to correct the error... discreetly! If you encounter any resistance, leave the clothing as it is. IT DOES NOT MATTER! Do not attempt to get the person to take the clothing off, turn it right side out, or fix it in any way. Taking off clothing that was just put on does not make sense to the person experiencing dementia. Your action only upsets the person and causes increased resistance. Later, when the moment seems appropriate, explain the clothing problem to the person. As a rule he will comply, and allow adjustments to his clothing. Alternatively, have someone else point out the difficulty. No arrangement or disarray of clothing is worth fighting over! Explain to staff members, families, VIPs, and visitors that the main goal is to keep the person with dementia feeling comfortable and in control. Occasional bizarre dress isn't important!

I REMEMBER SEEING *a staff member struggling with a man who was putting on a woman's sweater. He had one arm in the sleeve, and was determined to put that sweater on. The staff member tried just as determinedly to pull it off, explaining that it was not his sweater.*

The whole incident was escalating out of control, so I suggested we just leave him alone and watch what happened. The man marched off down the hall, pulling the very small sweater over his burly shoulders. Of course the sweater was very uncomfortable, pulling his arms back and constricting his movements, so after a few moments he pulled it off and tossed it on a chair in disgust. The staff member was then able to offer him his own sweater, and retrieve the discarded one for its proper owner.

If you don't insist, he won't resist.

—MARY LUCERNO, HEALTH EDUCATOR, FLORIDA

A HEAD NURSE TOLD ME *a wonderful story of a very influential businessman with Alzheimer's disease who lived in a Gentlecare unit. It was almost impossible to get him to change his clothing until the staff devised a terrific and effective strategy for doing so.*

One of them would approach the man and ask if he had any jobs available. The man invariably said he did, but the person would have to have an interview. So the "interview" would be set just after lunch. Another staff member would then approach the man and whisper to him, "You will want to have a fresh shirt and tie when you conduct that interview, won't you?" Without a murmur, the man would agree, have a bath, get dressed, and go off to have his lunch looking like a million dollars, pride intact. And of course, after lunch he would have forgotten all about the interview!

Like any other ADL, dressing is very personal and private. The more control we can give the person—even if it is only the illusion of control—the more pleasant and comfortable the activity will be. Experiment, modify, adapt, observe; and when you find something that works, tell everyone about it. Reinforcing a person's identity and well-being by taking time over dressing will influence his whole outlook for the rest of the day and make life much more pleasant for him, his family, and those of us who provide care.

Bathing

No ADL causes more distress or controversy than bathing. The deficits of dementing illness, in and of themselves, cause people to be fearful, anxious, angry, and confused about bathing—and therefore resistant to it. However, my experience leads me to believe that organizational and structural issues are the root of most problems surrounding bathing.

Current bathing practices in the long-term health care system are strongly driven by the biomedical model of care and its values: cleanliness, infection control, skin care, and predictable, efficient routine. Physical care preempts all other considerations. Consider the situation of an elderly man with dementia—possibly a man who was the owner of a company, the head of a large family, and an active member of his church and community—who has been scheduled for a bath at 10:30 on a Wednesday morning. He is approached by two young women who are strangers to him (if he has met them before, he has no memory of them). They ask him to take off his clothes and sit on a moveable chair. He is then covered with a sheet and propelled down a busy hallway to a large and often cold room filled with mechanical equipment and supplies. In the company of strangers he is lowered into a tub full of water, bathed, dressed, and returned to his room.

If this man resists these activities in any way, other staff members will be called to assist in restraining him. (I have seen as many as five staff people involved in bathing one person.) If the man's resistance to bathing persists, in future he will be given medication (a chemical restraint) before each scheduled bath time.

The procedure described here occurs, with variations, over and over again in long-term care facilities. It produces physically clean people, but at what cost? The psychological trauma to the person is severe, the stress and injury to staff is significant, and the distress of family caregivers is profound.

Obviously, people need to be bathed, and health care standards of cleanliness must be maintained. The challenge is to provide comforting, relaxed, stress-free bathing experiences for people with dementia without sacrificing personal control, dignity, privacy, and pleasure. Bathing should be a pleasurable experience!

Gentlecare research into bathing practices has taken us into hundreds of facilities and home care programs serving people with dementia in Canada, the United States, and Europe. In many facilities, bath time is the highlight of the day (or evening). In others, it is utter disaster. The different outcomes appear to result from the way the activity of bathing is perceived, and the way in which it is organized.

Bathing should be a pleasurable experience.

The Gentlecare bathing process is based on the successful experiences of care providers, and supports the belief that bathing is a powerful way to provide comfort and reduce stress. The Gentlecare formula is helpful in establishing a satisfying bath time routine. It reminds us to ask ourselves, as we are about to bathe someone—

- Who is this person?
- What is the disease process?
- What deficits does he have?
- What information does behavior provide?
- What prosthesis is required?

If we consider the socio-cultural aspects of bathing for the population of elders we care for, we must remember that many people in this generation—

- did not bathe daily, possibly not even weekly or monthly;
- did not often bathe immersed in water;
- never appeared nude before strangers or other family members;
- are frightened of water; and
- are not familiar with showers, mechanical lifts, Jacuzzis, etc.

MANY YEARS AGO I WORKED *in a hospital for elderly veterans. My colleagues and I had a very difficult time persuading these old gentlemen to have weekly baths. One man told me in no uncertain terms that he bathed once a year, in the spring. On that occasion, he cut off his combination underwear, had a bath, and put on his new under-wear for the coming year. No way was he going to take a bath "every five minutes!"*

With 200 reluctant bathers, the cleanliness issue was becoming so critical that we were forced to come up with a creative solution. So we introduced wrestling! Once a week we offered a program of wrestling, with beer and snacks in the auditorium. However, the price of admission was a detour through the showers. Each man was given clean clothes, nail care, haircuts, skin care, and a thorough shower. The program worked like magic, with long line-ups heading into the showers and exiting into the wrestling arena in the auditorium.

Gentlecare guidelines for bathing

Explain, explain, explain:
- Make sure the person with dementia understands the activity you are introducing. As we did with the veterans, give the person a reason to do what you want them to do, such as, "Your family is coming to visit"; "You'll want a bath before you get dressed up"; or "It's laundry day—I need your clothes for the washer" (this works for men).
- Avoid telling people they smell awful. This is insulting and causes elderly people who have lost their sense of smell to become defensive. Instead, use phrases like "freshening up," "feeling better," "nice and clean," "while the water's hot," "before all the water is used up," "this will help you sleep." And there's always the old standby: asking the person to help you in some way in the bathroom.
- Be sure the person understands who you are. Explain your role as a helper over and over and in a variety of ways throughout the bath. Try to blend into the activity, being as discreet as possible. Avoid giving orders or ultimatums, and listen to the tone of your own voice.

Prepare the environment:
- Bathrooms should look, feel, and smell like places where one would want to have a bath.

- Bathrooms should be warm and free of drafts.
- Limit the visual size of the room by using privacy curtains or screens.
- Avoid using the bathing area for storage of equipment and/or supplies, and thereby making it look like a warehouse.
- Remove posted literature from direct view of the client.
- Normalize the room with hanging plants, pictures, decorative towels, and bathroom objects.
- Warming closets for towels, flannel sheets, and robes adds a lovely touch. Using warm sheets at bedtime brings forth magical results.
- Ensure that the tub and toilet contrast with the floor and wall, with good figure/ground distinction. Camouflage all equipment, shelves, etc., not used by the person.

I MET AN OLD GENTLEMAN *I had helped, walking down the corridor of a facility. He was all disheveled and seemed upset. When I asked if something was the matter, he replied, "Oh! Moyra—I've just been through a car wash!"*

Post an "in-use" sign on the bathroom door, and limit traffic in and out of the room while it is in use:
- *Never* use the bathroom for more than one person at a time!
- While helping someone bathe, staff should not be required to address any other responsibilities, or take phone calls.

Avoid the use of mechanical equipment unless it is absolutely necessary:
- People experiencing dementia should use a regular bathtub for as long as possible.
- Avoid the use of a Jacuzzi unless the person is very comfortable with the sensation. Practice a desensitization process by having the person experience how the Jacuzzi works before using it. Remember that Jacuzzi use may not be a familiar activity for elderly people.
- Cover the inner surface of the regular tub with non-slip material.
- Use a low seat in a regular tub together with a hand-held showerhead.

- Position grab bars in the regular tub to promote maximum function. Avoid confusing the person with a maze of bars. Keep it simple but functional.

I REMEMBER WORKING *with a large man who was extremely resistant to bathing. Several staff people were always required to force him into the bath, and many of them had sustained injuries. As he hit out and screamed "Pig! Pig! Pig! Pig! Pig!" at everyone in the room, he clearly was a danger to anyone within his reach. We knew something about the bath was disturbing him and causing his violent resistance—but we didn't know what that something was.*

Always when we reach an impasse like this, it is important to examine our knowledge base. Using the Gentlecare formula, I decided to find out more about this man in order to understand his behavior. I met with the man's large, supportive family and discovered that he had been a farmer until he was hospitalized. Family members told me he was a gentle man who was always meticulous about his personal appearance and hygiene. I asked about his work, and his son told me he was a pig farmer. Hmmm...? So I asked about pig farming, and one of the things I was told was that after one killed a pig, one doused it in boiling water to remove the hairs. As the son mimed this activity for me, an image of his father tied in a chair and being lowered into the bubbling water of the Jacuzzi came vividly. Of course! Unfamiliar with a Jacuzzi and with limited vocabulary, the old gentleman had been trying desperately to tell us that we were going to scald him like a pig!

I returned to the facility with a new understanding of the person, and suggested that we offer him the opportunity to bathe in a regular tub. This he did, by himself, with a minimum of fuss or involvement by staff.

Think through the bathing process step by step to ensure that all the equipment and/or supplies needed are at hand:
- Prepare the bath area before you bring the person into the room.

- Ensure that an emergency call button is within reach of attending staff.
- If the person exhibits perceptual problems and appears not to be able to see the water, try adding food coloring to the water (use yellow, green or blue and avoid red).
- Try placing a flannel sheet or a heavy bath towel on the inside of a regular tub to avoid skin contact with the cool, slippery surface of the tub.
- Cover seats or lifts with towels before the person sits on them.
- Cover shower seats with a large, colorful bath towel.

Consider using bath teams:
Some people can give beautiful baths and others can't. Choose one or two caregivers who are particularly skilled in bathing and persuasion, and make them responsible for this activity (including the ambiance of the room and assembling necessary supplies and equipment). These people can also be responsible for skin inspection and care (lotion to hands, elbows, feet, and face), nail care, and assessment of general mobility.

Allow time for staff to assist with a relaxing, refreshing bath. Make bath time a significant treatment modality:
- Always give the person being bathed a "nutrition boost" before beginning the bath. Cheese and crackers, a peanut butter and jam sandwich, a muffin or a milk pudding, a shake or a smoothie—any of these can dramatically improve bath time.
- Avoid nudity. Always drape the person in towels throughout the bath.
- Make sure shoulders are covered.
- Place a towel over the lap.
- Some care providers use a towel that fastens around the waist or chest with Velcro and can be worn up to the point at which the person is submerged in water.
- If the person resists removal of a nightgown or pajama bottom, start the bath with the garment still on. The assisting staff can often slip the garment off without a fuss once it is wet.

- Never pour water over the head or face.
- Give lots of orienting information and encouragement.
- Always reward a successful bathing experience.

Arrange for flexible bathing schedules:
Some people prefer to bathe on awakening before they are dressed for the day. Others have traditionally bathed at night, before bedtime. Try to respect these lifelong habits. Determine the best time for a bath in consultation with the person, the family, and other caregivers. Make bathing a part of the individual treatment or care plan, rather than designating Wednesday or Thursday as bath day, and systematically bathing one person after another at 15-minute intervals whether they want to bathe or not. Remember that a sponge bath is always more effective than a fight over a tub bath. Sometimes it is possible to bathe only a part of the person before they stop cooperating. Never force a person to complete a bath! Do the best you can; then decide to try again at another time, or ask another caregiver to attempt to assist the person.

Consider using distractions:
- Always try to put an object between you, as assistant, and the person's body. For example, put the washcloth or showerhead in the person's hand, and then put your hand over the person's hand. This gives the illusion that the person is in control, rather than making them feel they are passively being bathed.
- Try back scrubs or massage to help the person relax into the bath before you begin bathing more intimate parts of the body.
- Give the person a drink or bite to eat at intervals during the bath.

ONE GENTLEMAN WAS IMPOSSIBLE *to bathe. I asked the staff if there was a favorite treat that he really loved. They said, yes, a bottle of beer. I said to the man, "Charlie, would you like a beer?" and he said, "Sure would!" I said, "As soon as we get you into the bathtub, I'll get a beer for you." The moment Charlie sat down in the tub I gave him his beer, which he drank with great enjoyment while we completed his bath. Now a bottle of beer signals a pleasant bath.*

Take advantage of bathing programs:

Bathing programs offered by day care services are invaluable for people living at home. Since most care in the home is provided by elderly female spouses, bathing is often exhausting and sometimes dangerous. Home support programs with access to facility bathing equipment are also an important aspect of dementia care. Often people with dementia resist having family members assist with their baths. Conversely, family carers may be the only ones who are allowed to help with bathing!

Mini-bath.

Install a mini-bath:

It is important to have regular bathtub facilities for general hygiene and relaxation, but mini-baths can reduce much of the fuss and bother associated with routine bathing. Special note: like ice cream, nobody does bathrooms better than Italians! In Italy it is common to see a mini-bath (not a bidet) located beside the toilet in each bathroom of a care facility.

A mini-bath is a small mesh chair that folds into the wall beside the toilet. Below it in the floor is a drain, and above it there is a hand-held shower head. Each morning the person being cared for is toileted, then shifted to the bath seat for bathing. Then the person is covered with a large, warm towel, groomed, and dressed. The process is so natural and efficient that the bath is simply considered a normal part of the day. The mini-bath is also highly effective for management of toileting accidents during the day or at night. Each bathroom also offers clean and dirty linen storage in the wall adjacent to the mini-bath—a wonderful feature!

Shower chair.

Mechanical bathtubs can often be frightening.

Eating

Eating is so important a core activity, such a powerful means of therapy in dementia care that in Gentlecare, we have devoted three separate chapters to this topic: Chapters 10, 11, and 12 discuss the role of nutrition in dementing illness.

Necessary Activities

FIGURE 9-6

Natural sleep, rest, relaxation, and privacy are activities necessary for human health. As people age, their sleeping patterns change dramatically. Older people seem to benefit from "power naps," and tend to sleep for shorter periods, and nap more frequently as their energy becomes depleted.

The process of living with dementia is exhausting. It is often hard to find a quiet opportunity to rest and regenerate. In addition, the dementing process causes older people to be confused between night and day (mind blindness), so they often sleep more during the day and wander around during the night.

Change in sleep patterns among elderly people is rarely considered in dementia care. It is not unusual to encounter the expectation that older people will stay in their beds for 12 hours or more—or contrariwise, stay out of their beds for 12 hours. This expectation, however convenient it may be for the system, runs counter to the knowledge that as they age, people sleep at night for shorter and shorter periods and nap more frequently during the day.

Gentlecare takes all these factors into account, arranging natural sleep periods that accommodate the older person's unique body rhythm. Programs and special quiet areas permit older people to get up in the night, receive refreshment, have socialization opportunities, and then often a return to sleep.

Natural sleep, rest, relaxation, and privacy are activities necessary for human health.

Exhaustion and resulting catastrophic behavior is prevented by building rest opportunities into each individual's care plan. Rest is prescribed between each complex undertaking—wake-up, rest, grooming, rest, dressing, rest, breakfast, rest, etc. Opportunities are also provided for elderly people to be alone, free of demands, and to have private spaces which they control. Necessary activities organized into the life of elderly people reduces fatigue, stree, catastrophic reactions, and gives the person energy to enjoy life.

Essential Activities

The activities of communication, movement, interaction with family, and intimacy are essential for human interaction. Dementia and standard dementia care rob elderly people of these vital life-enhancing activities. Essential activities woven into the lives of elderly people reduce stress and anxiety, and help them to enjoy life.

Communication

Communication is a human being's critical activity—it's what makes us different from other animals. Communication is a wonderful and complex activity. It involves talking and listening, and is verbal and non-verbal. Effective communication with people afflicted with dementia requires more than just talking. It requires preparation, knowledge, and new skills. But communication activities are worth the preparation since it is one of the loveliest activities you can do with elderly people. The following communication tips help us connect with elderly people:

- Establish who you are.
- Get permission to enter the person's space.
- Sit down, make eye contact.
- Focus or "ground" the person.
- Slow the pace and let the person set the pace.
- Take your time—make the time.
- Speak so the person can hear and see you.
- Be understandable and clear.
- Listen; remember that silence is golden.
- Be sensitive to feelings.
- Don't tease.
- Don't call them by "funny" names.
- Don't patronize.
- Minimize distraction.
- Use an object as an intermediary.
- Discuss whatever subject they suggest.
- Listen to the same old story as often as it is told.
- Express gratitude for the privilege, fun, experience, and honor of being there.

FIGURE 9-7

The following topics are communication strategies that work:

- "Remember when . . . stamps were two cents, eggs were ten cents a dozen . . . you bought your first car?"
- Talk about a subject through an object (perhaps something in the room).
- Don't ask questions. Give information instead.
- Don't ask, "How are you?
- Say: "You look nice/sleepy/lonesome/happy."
- "I like your sweater. It's a lovely color!"
- "Oh, I'm out of breath! Can I sit a minute with you?"
- Discuss family issues—theirs, yours, or the Queen's/famous people.
- Talk about what you saw on your way here to visit.
- Sports—especially good for men. Ask them to explain sports to you.
- Concerts/music—"I heard the loveliest _____!"
- "I would like to read to you. Would you like to listen?"
- War—medals and stories/church/prices and shopping/pets.
- The "old" days: their careers, different jobs, achievements—life review.
- Talk about dying: help them plan creatively; use your own feelings and experiences. Listen for: "I'm so tired of living. Everyone says I'm OK. I'm not OK."

Movement

Older people benefit greatly from the freedom to move indoors and outdoors spontaneously. For many this is a normal lifelong pattern of activity. Gentlecare emphasizes preparation of good walking spaces, accessible exits and entrances, and interesting activity that encourages movement through attractive settings and pleasing gardens. We emphasize music and dancing, working, playing with children, and helping activities . . . any activity that stimulates movement. We avoid artificial movement activities such as exercise groups that depend on staff to organize and initiate. Rather, we recommend spontaneous, on-

ACTIVITIES RELATED TO COMMUNICATION WHILE VISITING ELDERLY PEOPLE

- Explain and reassure them about current living arrangements.

- *If they ask*—reassure them about finances.

- Bring a bouquet of flowers and talk about them; arrange them together; look at them; hold and smell them.

- Bring a basket of objects as conversation pieces, then leave a pretty hankie, a piece of lace, a card.

- Help them write to friends and family.

- Help them record their life history.

- Bring a baby to visit.

- Bring a pet to visit.

- Find their favorite reading material and read aloud to them—the newspaper; *Reader's Digest,* etc.; the Bible or a daily meditation. Bring a selection of coffee table picture books and discuss them.

- Read the lyrics of songs.

- Read or recite familiar poetry, nursery rhymes together.

- Read inspirational material to them.

- Read old recipes and discuss them.

- Do gentle shoulder massage.

- Brush their hair.

- Massage their hands and feet with scented lotion. Manicure their nails.

- Bring a potted plant and discuss gardening.

- Bring colorful pictures of pets, kids, garden, and food.

- Wind wool with them.

- You do crafts while you visit and discuss.

- Take tiny gifts—three chocolates, soap, piece of costume jewelry, handkerchief, and samples of perfume.

- Unravel old knitting—a sweater—and discuss.

- Tear cloth for braided rugs. Show them a finished rug. Discuss.

- Have the person assist you with braiding.

- Promote bonding with another person nearby.

Through words, we actively construct our social world.

FIGURE 9-8

- Pray with them. Sing with them.

- Spend 5 to 10 minutes browsing through and discussing large picture books—barns, horses, gardens, embroidery, the Royal Family.

- Use old memory to help the person regain control—encourage communication using one of these ideas: pictures and photographs; babies and children; antiques to polish; reminiscing and story telling; pets (brought in by family or staff); familiar objects (lace, shells, buttons, beads and other jewelry); stamps; coins (collections); hats.

- Try to engage them in: WORK + TALK + REMEMBER!—sorting; cutting paper; folding, cutting up cards; putting paper in envelopes.

- Promote movement. Walk and talk.

- Bring a collection of hats to try on and talk about.

- Bring in an old-fashioned dress, a ball gown or wedding gown or kilt and talk about it.

- Bring in old carpentry and kitchen utensils and tools to talk about.

- Arrange for a roving troubadour to play a guitar, harp, mouth organ, or keyboard.

- Sing and hum favorite hymns and songs.

- Bring a Walkman with earphones.

- Talk about Dame Vera Lynn or some other famous singers and hum their hit tunes.

- Bring a tape and play one lovely piece.

- Have a hymn sing after supper, repeating first verses of familiar old hymns.

- Write letters for them to family members, friends, people within the facility including management (and they should answer!), the editor of local newspapers, the Queen, Prime Minister, MLA, Major, Senator, Congressman (they will answer).

- Set up a mail box.

- Deliver mail.

- Send mail to everyone in the care facility (this is an excellent activity for shut-ins, older volunteers to do); do all year round.

- Help them prepare a few Christmas cards for special friends and family.

—Some items adapted from *Aging is a Family Affair* by Wendy Thompson [Family Books, NC Press Ltd., 1990].

going familiar opportunities that elderly people can access on their own or with minimal help from volunteers, staff, or families.

As the diseases of dementia progress, many changes in motor function must be accommodated. Creative patterns of movement must be devised to maintain strength and flexibility. Gentlecare finds that familiar patterns of work often have the best chances of maintaining interest and involvement. For instance, an elderly lady will hang out laundry (upper arm movement) or fold children's clothing (manual dexterity) for long periods. They will only pull on a pulley a few times, and then only if a staff member is there to encourage them.

As the disease progresses, winding, tearing cloth or paper, bunching up paper, folding, braiding, unwinding knitting, and similar simple activities maintain upper arm strength. However, Gentlecare tries to keep everyone walking or dancing for as long as possible.

Intimacy/Touch

Dementia robs people of spontaneity—of the ability to reach out and connect with another human being socially or physically.

Gentlecare recommends using the power of touch to cut through this disease-induced barrier. We recommend activities such as massage of hands, feet, back, and head, hugs, dancing, hair brushing, manicures, pets, kids, and babies to help elderly people feel loved and included in the human family. Gentlecare encourages intimacy between spouses and arranges private spaces for them.

Often people afflicted with dementia mistake others for their spouse. If people with dementia bond, and no one is hurt or exploited, these relationships are supported. It is very important to discuss such activity with family members. However, regardless of the feelings of others, the person with dementia has the right to pursue relationships. Staff members need to monitor activity of this nature closely without judging or condemning. Gentlecare experience has shown that the more "legitimate intimacy" is introduced into regular programming, the less need there appears to be for sexual activity. It is not surprising that older people, like anyone, want to be loved and accepted.

Meaningful Activities

Work and leisure activities include special undertakings that require cognition, skills, and a great deal of support. On occasion, emphasizing overlearned, familiar areas of competency, Gentlecare finds that elderly people can achieve success at this level of function.

FIGURE 9-9

Good friends are a comfort.

WHILE WORKING IN A LONG-TERM *care facility, I particularly noticed an elderly man in a geriatric chair because he was very tall and appeared very uncomfortable. When I talked with him it was obvious that dementing illness had robbed him of significant function. However, he told me that he had operated a farm in the countryside of Ontario, Canada, and that he sold wood for a living. He was confined to the "geriatric" chair because he had a tendency to wander outdoors, and the facility on that day was short staffed.*

Since the man was perfectly fit physically, we devised a care plan for him that involved piling wood into a pile. This activity progressed very well with the elderly man piling the wood by day, and staff pulling the wood pile down by night. One day, however, he became very angry, complaining that "vandals" were messing with his wood pile. We had been caught! So we modified the plan, having the maintenance worker "buy" the completed pile of wood on the condition that the man throw it into the back of the truck. The maintenance staff would then drive off and return to dump a "new" load of wood to be piled. One day we looked out and discovered that the old gentleman was sitting on a stump of wood watching as two other men piled the wood!

ONE DAY, A VOLUNTEER *brought in a huge basket of fresh blackberries to a special care unit. But staff looked at it in dismay, not knowing what to do with this gift. An elderly lady classified as requiring total care with grooming and eating activities came into the kitchen and asked if she could make a pie since baking is such a complex ac-*

tivity. I considered the mess we might create, but thought to give it a try. So I put the necessary ingredients out in a row on the counter. With lightning speed, she whipped up the most delicious fruit pie any of us had ever tasted!

These stories illustrate the power of residual brain function, particularly if the person's long-standing areas of competency are stimulated and supported. Overlearned skills often remain functional even if the person cannot learn new skills, e.g., handshakes, opening doors for women, singing hymns, dancing, cleaning, etc. If staff are skilled and families are supportive, if environments feel like a familiar home, if activities mean something to elderly people, then on occasion magic happens. But it is important when working with people experiencing dementia to not hold out unreasonable hope that this level of achievement will occur routinely.

Meaningful activities require coordination of many levels of skills.

10
Rediscovering the Joy

Tell me—I'll forget
Show me—I may remember
But involve me, and I'll understand
—Ancient Chinese proverb

I gained valuable insights about dementia from watching my father dig holes in his lovely garden. At first, I was aghast as I watched the destruction. I had always regarded my father as a gardener, and I had a preconceived notion about how he should perform this activity. I could not accept my talented father operating at such a primitive level. I had to do something—draw the problem to his attention, show him how to do it, fix it for him, do it differently, make it turn out the way it was supposed to look!

I think I probably would have continued to think about activity for my father this way had I not been lucky enough at one moment to observe his face as he dug holes: he was as happy as he could be! He laughed and smiled occasionally, and focused on the task with such determination and joy that all the helplessness of dementia—the frustration, confusion, blundering, and ugliness—disappeared. This man was back in control, enjoying a feeling of accomplishment, reveling in an activity that made sense to him.

From that moment I abandoned any notions I had had of ever seeing my father perform at his previous level of functioning. I began to regard all activity as a series of tasks that could be simplified, modified, and broken into pieces that he could find achieveable. For instance, tasks could be shared. I could do the difficult parts and he could manage the simpler ones. If I were sufficiently clever and discreet, he'd never even know we weren't contributing to the task on an equal basis. As I learned more about the destruction taking place in his brain, I was able to devise more and more effective ways of engaging him in activities.

But no matter how creative I was, the activities that he thought up himself engaged him most completely and had the most healing effect. I grew skilled at watching him in action, discovering what it was he was attempting to do, and working along with him to achieve his desired goal.

When my father was involved in an activity of his own choosing, he was not angry or frustrated. He did not swear or throw things about; he was his usual pleasant self. As soon as we moved into an activity requiring me, my mother, or a staff member to be in control—giving instructions, rushing him along, expecting him to perform at levels no longer possible—then the fireworks began. After some weeks of experimentation, I learned to prepare for an activity by leaving objects, supplies, and tasks about for my father to discover on his own. Preparing in that way expanded the variety of things we could do, and gave us both great pleasure. My father liked to do sensible things, helpful things, and messy activities. He liked activities that required him to do the same thing over and over again, like stacking wood or raking leaves. He liked to be outdoors with his dogs. He liked to walk more than I did and watch other people talking and singing. And he loved to have people read to him.

And so I am indebted to my father for early and thorough training in dementia programming. Those experiments from long ago form the basis of the Powerpoint Program principles that we use in Gentlecare today.

Designing Powerpoint Programs
Using the 5+10 Formula

Activities for people with dementia can be viewed as simple and complex. *Simple* activities have only one step and are repetitive. Those with a physical component that are related to past life experiences and former life roles are recommended for people with dementia. *Complex* ac-

TEN STEPS THAT HELP A PERSON
WITH ACTIVITIES

1. Set the stage: remove distractions; be prepared; and choose an activity within the person's ability to perform.
2. Get the person's attention and agreement to participate before you start.
3. Identify the task.
4. Break the task into its simplest components.
5. Communicate clearly and frequently.
6. Help effectively: assist the person to accomplish the work, rather than doing the task yourself while the person watches.
7. Provide for rest breaks, and praise frequently. Give a nutritional boost during the activity.
8. Watch for fatigue and stress. If you notice signs of fatigue, stop immediately and remove the stressor.
9. Help the person have a successful closure of the activity even though a task is not completed.
10. Celebrate the experience, and praise and validate the effort.

FIGURE 10-1

tivities, in contrast, consist of several parts that must fit with one another in order for a task to be completed. They require new learning and sequencing and depend on abstract concepts. They frequently involve large groups of people and the use of complex equipment and supplies.

Complex activities usually challenge performance in ways that may not be possible for someone with dementia. Such activities are often noisy and confusing and contain an element of rush. As a rule, people with dementia find complex activities too difficult and stressful.

In Gentlecare we organize activities indicated by the person's care plan by using the Powerpoint 5+10 formula. The 15 activities included in the formula are programmed for each individual, and form the basis for each person's daily life. Successful activities for people with dementia are—

- Simple: requires no new learning and consists of one step only without sequencing.

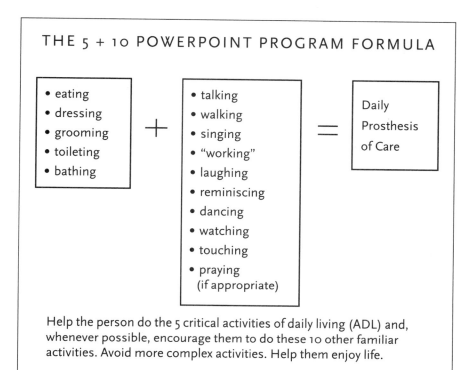

THE 5 + 10 POWERPOINT PROGRAM FORMULA

- eating
- dressing
- grooming
- toileting
- bathing

+

- talking
- walking
- singing
- "working"
- laughing
- reminiscing
- dancing
- watching
- touching
- praying
  (if appropriate)

=

Daily
Prosthesis
of Care

Help the person do the 5 critical activities of daily living (ADL) and, whenever possible, encourage them to do these 10 other familiar activities. Avoid more complex activities. Help them enjoy life.

FIGURE 10-2

- Personal: should provide something that the person with dementia can identify with, that means something to them.
- Realistic: an activity must be a task that "makes sense" to the person engaged in it. It helps if it is a useful activity.
- Stress-free: the activity must be "do-able," and the environment must be supportive.
- Happy and joyful. Programs should be fun.
- Successful: the person feels a sense of accomplishment.
- Energizing—not exhausting.
- Brief: lasts no more than 15 minutes, unless the person becomes engrossed in the activity.
- Familiar: based on former life skills, overlearned abilities.
- Functional: related to the person's own needs and life.
- Pertinent and necessary: baskets of peaches or tomatoes that must be used; guests who must be fed or served coffee: a bit of urgency makes the task exciting.

All activities mentioned in this book can be adapted for use at any point in the disease process. In the early stages of the disease, the person can be given greater responsibility, having more functional ability. In the middle stages of the illness, staff and family members need to offer more assistance or simplify the activity. In later stages of dementia, the person may be able only to assist, observe, or make marginal contributions to the activity. The activities indicated are adaptable for use in a person's home, in adult group homes, in assisted living programs, in nursing homes or long-term care facilities, in acute care hospitals, in palliative care situations, and in large psychiatric hospitals.

Dementing illness destroys people's ability to do things—certainly to do things at the level of performance that they formerly achieved. This presents an exceptional challenge for those of us who try to help them normalize their life in spite of dementia: how can we find appropriate, engaging activities that they can successfully carry out, in order to return meaning and satisfaction to their lives?

I have come to believe that the reason it is so difficult to arrange meaningful activities for these people is that we try too hard. We try to engage them in activities that look good, make a big impression, have a recognizable result, and make the person appear normal. We assign responsibility for activity to a few designated people in the organization when we know it takes all of us, families and volunteers included, to compensate for the effects of dementia. We fail to accurately assess and observe the people we work with to see what matters to them and what they are still capable of doing. We create environments devoid of materials or equipment that make normal activity possible. We think people with dementia cannot do anything—and sure enough, given our expectations, they can't!

It's time, long past time, to begin to relax and enjoy these wonderful elderly people. It's time we let them relax and enjoy a normal environment, filled with normal activities. It's time we let them fit in the best way they know how. When we begin to think differently about activity in dementia care, everyone wins.

GENTLECARE ACTIVITIES

These Work	These Don't
Validation: focusing on the person's legacy and accomplishments	Reality orientation
Reminiscing: joining their journey	Current event discussions/ quizzes
History maps: large posted maps of local areas with pictures of the person's farm, business, or home. Staff can draw the client's attention to them frequently.	
Role charts: jobs are assigned to each resident with titles attached. For example: Joe—floor cleaner; Molly—juice pourer. Contributions are acknowledged by all.	Bingo
Asset cards: 3 x 5 inch cards, prepared by the family, list interesting bits of information about the person (likes to play the mouth organ, etc.)	Card games/Puzzles
Letters and cards	
Hymn sings, war stories, folk songs, lullabies	
Just being in a garden, digging holes, sowing seeds, raking leaves, watering plants, picking flowers, fruit, or vegetables, eating garden produce	Gardening: this is a complex activity, which must be broken down into simple tasks (see list at left). Rules, sequences, specific procedures are too difficult for a person with Alzheimer's disease to accomodate.
Short car drives: in the early stages of the dementia process	Bus excursions: often result in relocation stress, anticipatory anxiety, and exhaustion

FIGURE 10-3

These Work	These Don't
Walking: indoors and outdoors	Aerobic exercises: those that require following directions and mirroring the activities of others
Dancing: with partners, line-dancing, or group dancing	
Marching	Circle groups (see above explanation)
Hugging: shoulder hugs work best	Ball toss: or any activity that involves tracking a moving object
Touching	
Handshakes and greetings	Sports: or any activity that requires sequencing or good hand/eye coordination
Laughing: at funny situations, costumes	
Massage: of hands, feet, back, shoulders	
Rocking chairs, gliders	Fire drills
Story telling	TV
Reading out loud: from Bibles, *Reader's Digest,* weather reports, recipes	Background music (Muzak)
	Stereo as background music or news
Old photo albums, large blow-ups of old photos	Public address systems
Slides: of family outings, animals, children	Large group activities
	Big entertainment groups
Small-group sing-songs, hymn sings	
Live music with one or two performers (roving troubadours)	
Dogs, cats, ducks, rabbits: all animals must be cared for by staff	Fish, birds: because they can't be touched and require a lot of care
Tasting food: ask a person's opinion; exchange recipes	

These Work	These Don't
Kneading: using pre-mixed dough (good for men)	
Watching cooking: men love to watch cooking, jam making, bread or pie baking	
Baking: prepared mixes, bread mix, making turkey stuffing	Baking: this is a complex task that must be broken down into simpler component parts
Stirring	
Scooping	
Rolling	
Decorating cookies, cake	
Folding, mending: children's clothing rather than towels	
Eating	
Serving	
Braiding, unraveling knitted goods	Crafts, making decorations
Tearing: paper, cloth	Pottery, ceramics
Cutting: paper, cloth	Sensory stimulation activities in kits, boxes, or put away in closets
Polishing: silver, copper, wood objects, jewelry	Aromatherapy in small containers
Moving: boxes, chairs, books	Taking part in organized events that the person must fit into and perform at predetermined levels
Dish washing, car washing: these activities have to be real and dramatic	
Dish drying	
Hand laundry	
Hanging out laundry on a clothesline	
Winding wool or cord	
Scrubbing	
"Helping" someone else	

These Work	These Don't
Rummaging: magazines, purses, old cards, hats, scarves, postcards, jewelry, little boxes; treasure chests filled with pictures, lace, buttons, shells, jewelry, hats, scarves, clothing; chests of drawers filled with treasures	Supplies locked in cupboards
Materials prepared for work activities like tidying, moving, packing in boxes, cleaning, washing	Activities that must be initiated and controlled by staff
Bookshelves with books and newspapers	Activities that are abstract (whose end products are not easily understood)
Cupboards with dishes/cutlery, produce	Activities that require sequencing, in which one part must be completed before the next part is undertaken
Hang on racks: rows of purses, aprons, hats, jewelry—as both wall decorations and enticements to activity; fill pockets with little treasures	Activities that stress order, cleanliness, tidiness

Gardening and yard work provide opportunities to do former favorite activities.

This lady was lonely until her "friend" came into her life.

Gardening is very complex so it is good when a friend helps out.

A dog is truly man's best friend.

Polishing a favorite saddle gives hours of pleasure.

Nothing makes people with dementia glow more than children.

A kitchen brings back wonderful memories.

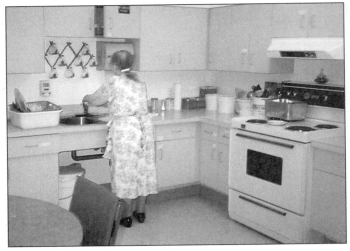

Comfort bags and purses provide safe places for treasures.

PART FOUR

NUTRITION IN DEMENTIA CARE

UNDERSTANDING
ALZHEIMER'S
DISEASE

PEOPLE
AND THEIR
IMPACT
ON CARE

ASSESSMENT
IN
DEMENTIA
CARE

GENTLECARE
The Prosthetic
Life Care System
for People with
Dementia

DESIGN
FOR
LIVING

A NEW
APPROACH
TO
PROGRAMS

NUTRITION
IN
DEMENTIA
CARE

11

The Act of Eating

(The nutritional material for the Gentlecare System has been developed in collaboration with Lorna L. Seaman, RPDT)

*All human history attests
that happiness for man
depends on dinner.*
—Lord Byron

Food is one of life's greatest pleasures, and no group of people appreciates meals more than elderly people. Mealtime, throughout history, in all parts of the world, has been a time for social interaction, a time to nourish ourselves, an occasion for celebration, a time to replenish our energy.

Eating is also one of the five major activities of daily living (ADLs), and possibly the most demanding.

Most of us take the act of eating for granted. We eat when we feel hungry. Apart from awareness of the pleasurable feeling provided by our taste senses, eating is an automatic process. We see food, take what we want, put it in our mouth, swallow it, and feel satisfied. We repeat this process at least three, and often many more, times each day. Our work activities are often structured around mealtimes, providing us with a time to satisfy our hunger, rest, and visit with friends before resuming our duties. But it's probably the meals associated with special occasions that stick in our memory: the birthdays, anniversaries, and get-togethers when food has provided the focal point. Many special events in the year have been linked to certain foods—the turkey at

Christmas, the pumpkin pie at Thanksgiving. Each cultural group has developed its own special foods for times of celebration.

The food we eat so automatically is essential for life. Every one of the million living cells within the body needs energy to function—energy that is provided by the food we eat. Each cell in our body is a complex biomedical factory that must be supplied with its food energy in a precise form to function, so that all our cells can manage the myriad complex activities of daily living.

Aging and certain diseases that afflict older people can significantly change the experience of eating, affecting both the enjoyment and the nutritional benefits of food. Changes in vision, physical mobility, and the senses of taste and smell, to name only a few, affect the older person's ability to enjoy this most basic life-enhancing activity. Impediments to eating properly—that is, eating the right types of food in the right amounts at appropriate intervals—can dramatically affect both health and quality of life. For example—

- Significant numbers of older people suffer from *dysphagia* (difficulty in swallowing).
- In addition, the aging process affects dentition: 50 percent of people have no teeth by age 65; 67 percent have no teeth by age 75. Most people compensate for this problem by using dentures; however, when people are cognitively impaired, management of dentures becomes a challenge.
- As people age, the muscles necessary for chewing lose strength. Eating becomes more difficult and requires more energy. It is harder to control liquids as the tongue, cheeks, and lips become weaker. These difficulties can be made worse by the use of certain drugs.
- Also, the production of saliva (xerostomia) is reduced as people age. This decreases the effectiveness of the digestive process, the transportation of food, and the adhesion of dentures to the gums. Saliva production is, of course, affected by the use of drugs, and by warm environments.
- There is a 60-percent reduction in the number of taste buds on the

tongue as people age. After age 60, therefore, the sense of taste is less acute, and there is a consequent loss of enjoyment of eating and appetite. In addition to registering taste sensations (sweet, sour, salty, and bitter), the tongue is responsible both for moving food toward the stomach and for cleaning the mouth, and the effectiveness of these functions is diminished with age.

- With aging, there are marked changes in the sensations of smell, taste, and touch, together with a reduction in the cough reflex. These changes lead to increased incidents of aspiration of food and liquid by elderly people, which can result in pneumonia and even death.

- The sense of smell is registered in the limbic system of the brain *(rhinencephalon)*, which is significantly damaged by dementing illnesses. The sense of taste is made up of sensations from the mouth, which are interpreted jointly by the sensory cortex of the brain and the thalamus—both of which are damaged early in Alzheimer's disease.

- Aging affects vision and perception, making it difficult for older people to distinguish the presence of food on dishes, to differentiate among food types, and to use utensils efficiently in picking up food.

- Finally, it is estimated that the efficiency of metabolic processes is diminished by up to 20 percent as people age. Kidney function can be diminished by half, highlighting the critical issue of dehydration, and the importance of hydration programs. The excessive use of medication by elderly people can seriously exacerbate metabolic problems.

The changes due to aging alone are a sufficient challenge to good nutrition. However, three out of four elderly persons receiving health care services will also experience dementing illness. Significant numbers of them will suffer from another form of mental illness, such as depression. The impact on eating of this complex combination of problems requires a fresh new look at the role of nutrition in the care of elderly people.

Nutrition management is, therefore, a major dementia frontier. The dysfunction caused by dementia profoundly affects the eating process. As a result, the energy needed by the afflicted person for the performance of the complex tasks of daily living is severely compromised. In Gentlecare, we believe this energy drain is a major contributing factor in incidents of catastrophic behavior. People with dementing illnesses live in a world of anxiety, frustration, and fear. Such psychological chaos depletes energy, and if this is not replaced through good nutrition, people become defenceless in dealing with encroaching stress and turmoil.

Specific dysfunction such as *agnosia* (the inability to recognize familiar sensory stimuli) and *apraxia* (the inability to initiate purposeful movement) make it difficult for people with dementia to access their food. Conditions such as *bulimia* (in which people gorge themselves) make it impossible for them to monitor their food intake. When these problems are combined with loss of memory and degradation of the senses of taste and smell, it is little wonder that malnutrition can occur.

With malnutrition comes an exacerbation of all physical problems, together with the possibility of an *acute dementia,* the symptoms of which can mimic Alzheimer's disease. Distinguishing between an acute dementia (such as those caused by malnutrition or dehydration) and Alzheimer's disease requires careful and continuous assessment; if the condition proves to be acute dementia, the cause of the symptoms must then be addressed.

Dehydration directly affects the quality of elderly people's lives. Measuring appropriate water intake is problematic: How often have liquids been given? By whom? How much was actually consumed? Often elderly people cannot indicate that they are thirsty, so the assumption on the part of caregivers must always be that they need water or other liquids.

Eating is so automatic for most of us that it's hard to imagine the complexity of the process. If we hope to help older people with their meals, we need to be aware of the various stages in the act of eating.

It is very important to remember that a diet adapted to the client's condition is of no value unless it is eaten.

—DARLENE WEGER, CAREWEST, CALGARY, ALBERTA, CANADA

The Act of Eating

First Cognitive Stage

- The person who is eating must be aware of the activity taking place. Orienting information must be given frequently.
- The ambiance in the dining room must reflect the purpose of the room.
- The person must be willing to participate in the activity of eating. However, appetite may be reduced; there may be discomfort in eating with a large crowd; or there may be a sense of inability to afford to go into such a big restaurant.
- The person must agree to accept external aid. A bond or relationship needs to exist between the person eating and the person helping.
- The person who is eating must feel comfortable and secure, and must be allowed sufficient time to participate in and enjoy the activity.

SWALLOWING

The act of swallowing requires coordination of several nerves, 26 muscles of the mouth, the pharynx and esophagus, and the ability of the mind to focus on the activity.

Preparatory Stage

- The person's mouth and teeth should be clean, and dentures (if used) should be in place.
- Check to ensure that the person has no mouth pain or discomfort.

Try sitting on a low chair at a high table to personally experience how frustrating this can be.

Ensure that the person is in a comfortable, functional position, with his head in a neutral position or tilted forward and slightly downward: eating occurs in a flexion position.

Chairs that are too low or tables that are too high cause the person to stretch into an extension position, or to strain to raise his arms high enough to reach items on the table. Over time, this will cause exhaustion, which is a significant contributor to giving up on independent eating and requiring assistance at meals.

Ensure that each individual has cutlery and utensils appropriate to the specific level of function. Where appropriate, try the following:

- Use plates with lips.
- Use sectioned plates.
- Try using bowls instead of plates.
- Build up the handles of cutlery to permit a better grip.
- Use glasses with wide openings.
- Experiment with cups with wide openings and covers.
- Serve liquids in cups or mugs with large protruding handles.
- Use rubber-coated children's silverware for people who bite down on utensils.
- Use plain, solid dishes with curved edges.
- Ensure a good contrast between table or placemat and plate, and between plate and food items.

GENTLECARE Practice Tip

Check each chair and table for an effective functional relationship. Assess each individual to ensure that arms and shoulders clear the tabletop easily, and that all items are within easy reach. Place foam boosters under small or short people, and stools under their feet.

Oral Stage

- The food is chewed and mixed with saliva.
- The tongue gathers up food from around the mouth, teeth, and gums.
- The food is formed into a bolus at the tip of the tongue.
- The lips close and the cheeks tighten.
- The tongue squeezes the bolus against the hard palate.
- The food bolus is propelled toward the pharynx.
- The swallowing reflex is triggered.

Pharyngeal Stage

As this stage of eating—
- Respiration is temporarily halted.
- The epiglottis (the cartilage that covers the opening of the larynx) closes.
- The food bolus moves from the mouth into the esophagus by the process of *peristalsis* (contractions and relaxations of the muscular walls of the digestive tract).

GENTLECARE Practice Tip

Before you feed anyone one more bite of food, take a mouthful of your favorite food and work it through the seven stages of eating. This exercise will help you understand how difficult mealtime is for people experiencing dementia, and how much time it takes to eat a meal.

Esophageal Stage
- The food bolus is propelled toward the stomach.

Preparation Stage for Digestion

Once swallowing is accomplished, Gentlecare recommends the following strategies to assist in effective digestion:
- The person maintains a comfortable upright position for at least half an hour; or
- The person is involved in a gentle walking program.

Cognitive Stage for Digestion
- Avoid rush, noise, or confusion.
- Do not involve the person who has just eaten in any complex activity.
- Reduce stress of any kind. Rest for one additional hour after meals.

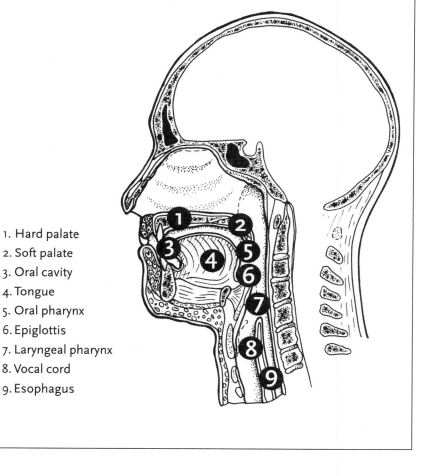

THE PHYSIOLOGY OF THE SWALLOWING PROCESS

1. Hard palate
2. Soft palate
3. Oral cavity
4. Tongue
5. Oral pharynx
6. Epiglottis
7. Laryngeal pharynx
8. Vocal cord
9. Esophagus

FIGURE 11-1

It is estimated that the average length of time allotted for meal consumption in long-term care facilities is 13 minutes. There is often a great rush to clean up dining rooms after meals and return dishes and utensils to the kitchen. Not infrequently, people are rushed through meals to accommodate the working schedules of food service and housekeeping staff. It is essential that all personnel understand how important and difficult mealtimes are for people with dementia. Staff need to be allocated sufficient time to carry out necessary cleaning tasks without cutting into residents' meal time.

Tips for Safe Swallowing

Assessment

Each person should have had an appropriate disease assessment and an assessment of functional abilities.

Positioning

The person eating should be seated upright, with his head slightly flexed forward. If the person is eating while in bed, ensure that head and shoulders are supported at an angle of no less than 60 degrees.

Presentation of Food

- Use a metal spoon, not plastic, or syringes, straws.
- Offer only one teaspoonful at a time.
- Allow sufficient time to chew and swallow.
- Watch for successful swallowing, food drooling out of mouth, coughing, or choking.
- Do not offer additional food unless food has been swallowed successfully.

Coughing/Choking

When a coughing episode begins, the individual should bend forward at the waist and lower his chin to his chest. Do not cover mouth with cloth or napkin. The force of the cough will clear the airway, and the position of the larynx will protect the airway from being reinvaded. Do not interfere unless the food becomes lodged in the larynx and the person cannot breathe. Then the Heimlich manoeuver should be performed.

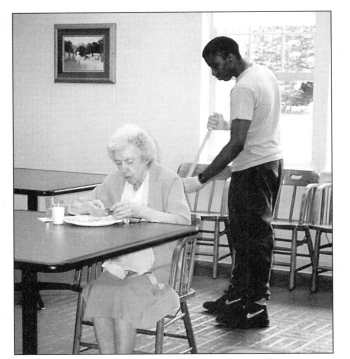

In some facilities, housekeeping staff are encouraged to work around people as they would in their own home.

To carry out the Heimlich manoeuver, approach the choking person from behind; reach around the person's body and lock your hands just below the rib cage. Give quick upward and backward jerks to the diaphragm. This provides a blast of air through the vocal cords (airway) which may blow out the obstruction. Refer to policy and procedures of individual institutions for specific strategies.

—Speech Language Pathology Department
Calgary District Hospital Group
Alberta, Canada

A human being swallows about 600 times each day...350 times while awake, 200 times while eating, and 50 times while sleeping.

12

Nutrition for Energy and Performance

It's good food and not fine words
that keep me alive.
—Molière

Gentlecare has developed a nutrition management process to help care providers organize all the various data and strategies about eating. The result is a workable formula that enables elderly people with dementing illnesses to consume the nutrients necessary for healthy living. The management process is called the Gentlecare Quality Management Cycle for Geriatric Nutrition Care.

The Management Cycle for Geriatric Nutrition Care

The long-term goal of the management cycle is the development of a complete personal nutrition plan; this requires completion of all of the steps of the cycle. However, any of the steps in the plan can be carried out individually, to the benefit of the person with dementia.

The cycle can begin at any point, but is usually started by creating a personal profile, which addresses the personal and cognitive aspects of nutritional assessment. The personal profile is recorded on the nutritional assessment form.

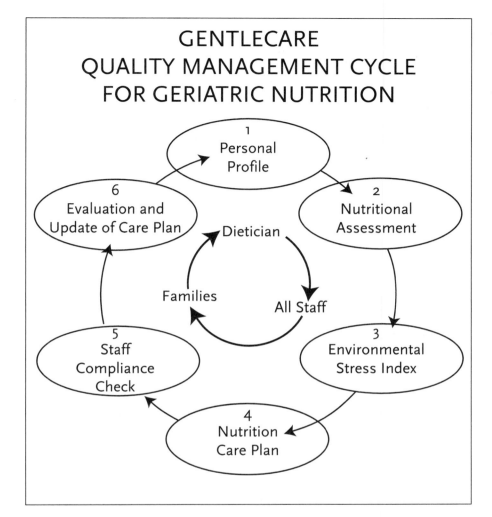

GENTLECARE
QUALITY MANAGEMENT CYCLE
FOR GERIATRIC NUTRITION

1
Personal
Profile

6
Evaluation and
Update of Care Plan

Dietician

2
Nutritional
Assessment

Families

All Staff

5
Staff
Compliance
Check

3
Environmental
Stress Index

4
Nutrition
Care Plan

FIGURE 12-1

Step 1: Personal Profile

DIAGNOSIS/MEDICAL HISTORY

To assess nutritional needs, a diagnosis of the illness(es) affecting the person must be established. Dementing illness causes the following deficits, which interfere with eating:

- altered consciousness (inability to process information)
- distractability
- poor judgement
- decreased awareness of people, place, and time
- decreased mobility/muscle coordination (apraxia)

- altered vision
- altered hearing
- poor appetite/excessive appetite
- lack of feeling in mouth
- diminished sense of taste and smell
- lack of ability to distinguish between food and other substances

FIGURE 12-2

STAGES OF THE DISEASE

Accelerated metabolism and activity in the early stages of dementing disease often result in weight loss. People so affected require greater than normal amounts of food to maintain energy and performance. If this need is not recognized, they may not be getting enough food.

Weight loss may be also be due to a number of factors, including—

- the stress of relocating from the family home
- unfamiliar foods
- confusing and/or frightening eating situations
- the expenditure of large amounts of energy in walking, due to anxiety, agitation, and night waking

As the disease progresses, people experiencing dementia lose the function of the hypothalamic center of the brain, which controls appetite. At that point, people may binge on food and gain weight. This is not because they have suddenly become greedy or gluttonous; rather, it is a side effect of dementia.

In the final stages of the disease, the dementing process accelerates and body mass is lost. No amount of supplementary or artificial feeding can reverse this phenomenon.

FAMILY/SOCIAL/CULTURAL INFORMATION

Family members can contribute essential information regarding food preferences and idiosyncrasies; they can also provide information about cultural food practices. Their contribution is an integral part of the nutrition care plan.

I WAS ONCE ASKED FOR ADVICE *regarding a woman who simply would not settle down at bedtime. The staff had tried everything, to no avail.*

Whenever I reach a stalemate in problem-solving, I always consult with family members—in this case, a large and caring Norwegian family. In the course of our discussion one niece said, "I don't know why Aunt Erna is causing so much trouble at bedtime. When I stayed with her in Oslo while I was going to university, every night we would sit and talk, have our warm milk and eels, and then she'd go straight to bed!"

And guess what? As soon as we had rustled up some eels and warm milk for her, we had no further problems.

Tell me what you eat and
I'll tell you what you are.

—ANSELME BRILLAT-
SAVARIN

ENERGY EXPENDITURE

Energy expenditure refers to the amount of energy needed by a person with dementia. This can vary over time, as can the amount of fluid needed and the amount of protein required to maintain health.

Energy requirements: recommended energy intake for a 75+ male is 2000 calories (add 600 calories if active). The recommended energy intake for a 75+ female is 1500 calories (add 600 calories if active).

Fluid requirement: 1 ml per 1 calorie intake.

Protein requirement: 1 gm per kilogram of body weight.

FIGURE 12-3

Note that the Gentlecare nutrition plan recommends an additional 600 calories (or portion thereof) for both men and women during those stages of the disease during which they are very active. This extra nutrition can be given in the form of nutrition boosts: protein drinks, smoothies, egg nogs, and other delicious nutritious supplements. Often family members will gladly supply these special nutrients if only they are asked. Gentlecare recommends trying a sports bottle to facilitate this mini-meal.

PREFERRED MEAL PATTERNS (TIMES AND FOODS)
Family advice and experimentation provide the necessary information on the best times for meals and snacks. This is one of the simplest and most effective strategies for reducing problematic behavior.

FIGURE 12-4

All sorrows are less
with bread.

—MIGUEL CERVANTES

Step 2: *Nutritional Assessment*

The next step in the cycle is the nutrition assessment, a process that screens for factors that affect the physiological aspects of nutrition. Every individual should be screened for:

EATING FUNCTION

SWALLOWING FUNCTION

Difficulties associated with swallowing:
It is important to note that one swallowing or choking incident, no matter how frightening, does not represent dysphagia. Effective assessment will determine whether the choking was physiological, due to cognitive dysfunction, or caused by poor feeding techniques, poor positioning, seating, or stress.

PHYSICAL DISABILITIES

The person being cared for must be checked to see that no physical disabilities exist that might interfere with nutritional status. For example, is the person able to function independently for eating?

- Sensory integration deficits in vision, hearing, perception, taste, or smell are noted;
- Laboratory data must establish possible problems;
- Fluid intake/hydration status must be monitored;
- Records of food intake and weight history are important;
- Therapeutic diet orders must be appropriate and up-to-date;
- Medications must be reviewed for possible effects on nutritional status;
- Nutrition-related problems should be reviewed, such as constipation, skin integrity, nausea, or vomiting;
- The possibility of pain interfering with eating should be investigated;
- Musculo-skeletal problems that might interfere with eating should be investigated.

Assessment of this data will help care providers define the person's level of nutritional risk. In Gentlecare the person's level of risk is measured not only by physical status, but also by cognitive abilities, leading to a much more effective assessment process. (See chart on Nutritional Risk Factors.)

CLASSIFICATION OF NUTRITIONAL RISK

COGNITIVE RISK FACTORS	PHYSIOLOGICAL RISK FACTORS

LOW RISK

early evidence of: • memory loss • disorientation to time and place • confusion • distractability • hyperactivity • alteration in appetite, thirst control mechanism • alterations in perception of sensory stimulation • heightened sensitivity to stimulation	• no recent significant weight change (10% in six months, 5% in one month) • eats independently • able to ambulate, sit at table • consumes most of food and fluid at each meal with regular utensils and dishes • consumes a variety of food types and textures from all food groups

MEDIUM RISK

• increased memory loss • no sense of time • increased confusion • loss of orientation to place • visual field neglect • inability to read • minimal to moderate evidence of agnosia, abulia, aphasia, anomia, and apraxia	• food allergies • chewing/swallowing difficulties • needs prosthetic aids for eating • chronic constipation • chronic or episodic diarrhea • persistent nausea or vomiting • post-gastrectomy dumping syndrome • weight loss or gain (of 10% of usual weight over six months) • poor or changed appetite • poor fluid intake • diabetes mellitus, non-insulin dependent • lactose intolerance • hypertension • trauma due to surgery • chronic infections (urinary tract infections, recurrent pneumonias)

HIGH RISK

• progression of all of the above • inability to initiate movement • increased difficulty swallowing	• unplanned weight loss (>5% in one month) • dysphasia, dehydration • diabetes mellitus, insulin-dependent • chronic or acute renal failure • severe decubitus ulcers or other open lesions • evidence of gastrointestinal bleeding, haematemesis, blood in the stool • total inability to move voluntarily • all systems closing down

FIGURE 12-5

Indicators of possible nutritional deficiencies in older adults include—

- pain or discomfort during or following eating
- a burning sensation while eating
- "pins and needles" or cramps in the legs
- loss of the sense of taste or smell
- weight loss or weight gain
- sore lips, tongue, or throat
- hair loss
- loss of appetite
- thin nails
- change in bowel habits
- regurgitation of food
- vomiting
- rash of dermatitis that does not respond to topical medication
- diarrhea
- blood in the stool
- bleeding patches on the skin or easy bruising
- light sensitivity
- slow healing of sores or ulcers
- swelling of the legs
- loss of balance
- changes in skin color (yellow, brown, or gray tinge to the skin)
- confusion
- depression
- breathlessness on exertion and/or while at rest

The Gentlecare Hydration Program

Dehydration is the cause of one of the acute dementias. Lack of water can cause problems similar to those seen in Alzheimer's disease. Furthermore, people with dementia can't always recognize thirst or ask for a drink if they feel thirsty, so the important task of monitoring their liquid intake must be undertaken by others. Therefore the companion-piece to the caloric intake of elderly people is a hydration program for each individual in care.

THIRST

- Thirst is a signal designed to prevent serious dehydration.
- The part of the brain that controls thirst is the limbic system.
- As the disease progresses and affects the hypothalmus, the person may suffer from a sensation of excessive thirst.
- Other deficits in the brain's function may result in the inability to articulate the need for fluids.
- Thus, it is possible that part of wandering, lethargic, irritable, and confused behaviors can be attributed to unsatisfied sensations of thirst and/or actual dehydration.
- Therefore, provision of adequate fluids when desired and in response to behavioral signals is a high priority.
- An effort to reduce incontinence with the restriction of fluids may result in dehydration, and in fact achieve the opposite of what was intended.

FIGURE 12-6

SIGNS OF DEHYDRATION

- fatigue
- confusion
- IRRITABILITY
- dizziness
- headaches
- low energy
- dry mouth
- dry skin
- loose, wrinkled skin
- sunken eyes
- low urine output (less than two cups)
- weakened muscles leading to falls

FIGURE 12-7

It's important to recognize the signs of dehydration.

DEHYDRATION FACTS

- The average body contains 40–50 quarts of water.
- A loss of 5 percent or 2½ quarts results in symptoms of dehydration.
- The body needs additional water to make up for losses to the air in dry, heated buildings.

• The daily water requirement is one milliliter for every calorie consumed, or 1500 milliliters or six cups for an intake of 1500 calories.

Remember that handing someone a glass of water only counts if the person drinks the glass of water! Many facilities have bottled water available in a central location; everyone who provides care should make it a practice to offer people water at every opportunity: whenever you see them, stop to talk with them, begin or end an intervention, at the start and end of programs, during meals, and during social events. Hydration is a vital part of the total nutrition program.

A small minority of people cannot drink water, while some elderly people simply don't enjoy drinking water, especially cold water. Special arrangements must be made in those cases. Gentlecare suggests the following substitutes:
- fruit juice popsicles
- pudding popsicles
- Jell-O popsicles
- freezies
- fruits (melon, pears, raspberies)
- soups
- canterbury tea (hot water with milk and sugar)
- lemonade
- sherbets

Liquids can be presented in a sports bottle. This often works for men. Avoid styrofoam cups.

Regular water intake should always be charted. The offer of water, and the monitoring of actual water intake, provides a perfect time for a brief communication, touch, hug, or a walk.

Incontinence

Incontinence is an enormous problem in dementia care—for the person with dementia, for families, and for staff. There is a myth that the more a person drinks, the more incontinent that person will be. Not so! In fact, regular hydration programs actually reduce incontinence and

UNDERSTANDING AND PREVENTING
INCONTINENCE

STANDARD CARE

Less fluid intake

Dehydration

Body conserves
fluids

Fluid retention

Increased fluid
pressure

Urge to urinate

Incontinence

GENTLECARE

More fluid intake

Hydration

Less fluid
retention

Normal excretion

Fewer urges
to urinate

Reduced
Incontinence

FIGURE 12-8

promote all-around better health and performance. This seeming paradox really has quite a simple explanation: when fluid intake is reduced, the result is dehydration. Recognizing that this is a problem, the body responds by retaining fluids. The retained fluids increase fluid pressure, which leads to a more frequent urge to urinate, and often to incontinence.

Conversely, if fluid intake is increased, the adequacy of hydration permits the body to release all excess fluid, without a defensive build-up of fluids. With a decrease in fluid retention, there is a lower frequency of the urge to urinate, and thus a decrease in incontinence.

Medications Can Affect Eating

Be aware that *neuroleptic* or *psychotropic* medications can be the cause of swallowing problems in significant numbers of the aged population. Thus their effects must be assessed very thoroughly with the pharmacist or physician.

Antidepressants, anti-psychotics, sedatives, and other similar drugs can cause dry mouth, reduced motor coordination, extra-pyramidal side effects, sedation, inattention, and drooling—all of which can affect the swallowing function.

The side effects of *anticholinergic* medication—decreased appetite, nausea, and vomiting—can seriously compromise food intake.

Many drugs, when taken over a long period, can produce vitamin and mineral deficiencies in the elderly that may severely compromise nutritional status and result in decreased general health and resistance to disease. Consequently, it is important to encourage a regular review of medications if a deterioration of health status is suspected to be a result of an iatrogenic (medication-related) condition.

Step 3: Environmental Stressors that Affect Eating

The next step in the management cycle is an assessment of environmental stress: an evaluation of the stress factors present in the macroenvironment. Data on stress is obtained by examining the following factors:

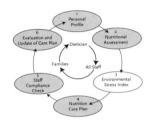

FIGURE 12-9

BEHAVIORAL MAPPING

Behavioral mapping is a technique whereby care staff observe and document the person with dementia over a 24-hour period. Some difficult situations may require a second 24-hour observation period. The person's behavior within the environmental context is observed, together with the nature of ongoing activities, interactions with others, and such physical factors as location, noise levels, and lighting quality. A study of these observational records can indicate the nature of environmental stressors; the timing of their occurrence; their behavioral consequences; and the schedules and personnel involved in the situation. (Fig. 7.5 p.104)

SUNDOWN SYNDROME

In people with dementia, there appears to be a correlation between times of performance expectation, accumulated stress, and catastrophic behaviors. A common instance is late afternoon "sundowning," which occurs when people with cognitive impairment seem to hit a low point and cannot summon the energy to manage daily life appropriately. At that point, any performance expectation placed upon them can cause them to go out of control.

Sundown syndrome may be attributed to the following factors:

- fatigue;
- lack of support during shift change and preparations for dinner;
- lack of light in the environment;
- drop in metabolism;
- pain; and
- other factors.

The catastrophic behavior can be ameliorated by the following interventions:

- frequent rest and naps;
- a support program of music, reading, massage, etc., in late afternoon or early evening;
- improved lighting in late afternoon;
- a nutrition boost mid- and late afternoon; and
- pain assessment and management.

THE EATING ENVIRONMENT

Factors to be evaluated for individual needs are the size of the room in which meals are served; the number of people dining; the level of noise; the appropriateness of the furniture; lighting quality; glare; heating; and seating arrangements must be evaluated in terms of their "match" to the needs of a given individual.

SYSTEM CHANGES

Effective nutritional care begins with changing the way we think about and implement meals for people experiencing dementia. Significant system and environmental changes will be needed if we are to enhance nutritional opportunities and decrease progressive dysfunction, excessive disability, and escalating costs. These changes include the following:

- Designate a specific dining area for people with dementia.
- Separate people in the dining area by their levels of dysfunction and cognition.
- Relax rigid mealtime schedules to allow sufficient time for the person with dementia to function or to be properly assisted. This is especially critical during the breakfast period.

- Ensure that all assisting personnel are skilled in evaluating dementia dysfunction, offering assistance, and reducing stress.

ENVIRONMENTAL INFLUENCES

- Ensure that the person with dementia understands that at mealtime, the appropriate activity is eating. This information may need to be repeated, and projected in several ways; for example, dining areas should look, smell, and feel like places one would want to eat in.

- Avoid presentation of food on trays. Loss of visual identification, smell, taste, and motor coordination makes it impossible for a person with dementia to understand that the tray contains a meal.

- Dining areas should be small, quiet, comfortable, and stress-free. Large dining areas should be subdivided to reduce confusion; half-walls and planters are useful in this regard.

- Lighting should allow people to see food items and the persons who are assisting them; therefore, light levels should be three times normal amounts. Lighting materials and floor finish should be arranged to avoid glare.

- Ventilation and heat control should provide a comfortable ambiance.

- Because eating is a complex task requiring great concentration, eliminate distractions, such as noises; TV; loud music; loud personal conversations between staff members; special entertainment during the actual meal hour (use music before or after meals but not during); doctors' rounds in the dining room during mealtime; and the distribution of medications at mealtime.

CURRENT MEAL PATTERN

The following factors must be reviewed in terms of each individual's former life patterns: flexibility of scheduling; time of meals; period of time allowed

After a good dinner, one can forgive anybody, even one's own relations.

—OSCAR WILDE

Contrast the visual information available to the person with dementia in these two dining rooms.

for eating meals; wake-up times; time spacing between meals; amounts of food served at each meal; and opportunities for rest after meals.

STRESS PROFILE

Using the data collected in the environmental stress assessment, an individual's stress levels are charted over a 24-hour period. The activities or factors that caused the individual to exceed the stress threshold can then be identified and appropriate changes made. (Fig. 7.3, p. 102)

INFLUENCE OF STAFF AND FAMILY MEMBERS

Assisting a person with dementia in eating is a challenging task requiring knowledge, skill, and patience. Being fed is a most unpleasant experience for adults. Gentlecare recommends that anyone who undertakes the task of feeding another person should experience being fed firsthand. And staff needs to be allocated appropriate amounts of time to help people with their meals. Pacing, communication, and physical interaction between residents and assisting personnel must be regularly monitored and assessed.

Gentlecare believes strongly in involving family members at mealtimes to normalize the experience of eating and enhance social interaction. However, family members may need help in learning how to assist people appropriately. Families are under stress when caring for their loved ones; they may demand a level of performance that the person being cared for can no longer achieve. They may over-help, or over-feed; they may be too talkative or provide too much distraction. As a result, their presence may cause anxiety.

Almost without exception, family members feel guilty about having their loved ones in an institution. No matter how often they are reassured that there is no basis for this feeling, guilt happens. In our society, one of the common ways we relieve guilt is by offering food. Sometimes, homemade food can really brighten a person's day. On the other hand, food may be offered at inappropriate times or in inappropriate ways, so staff and families need to strike a balance that works for the afflicted person.

It should be noted that on occasion family members eat food provided for the person with dementia, especially if that person does not seem to want the meal. Gentlecare recommends that family members be encouraged to join their relatives for meals rather than be asked or expected to "come in and feed your mother." People with dementia are more likely to eat at meals if others around them are eating as well. The cost of providing family members with meals is minimal compared to the therapeutic value of the family presence. If budgets are a problem, offer beverages only or beverages and dessert.

We recommend a modified practice for staff members, encouraging them to carry a cup of coffee or tea with them to give the illusion of joining with residents in the meal. This practice normalizes the meal and diminishes the perception that staff members are waiters.

Step 4: The Development of a Nutrition Care Plan

The next step in the management cycle is the development of a Nutrition Care Plan.

The accumulated data of the personal profile, the nutrition assessment, and the environmental stress index is collected by the dietician, assisted by members of the interdisciplinary care team. This data is then tested against the Gentlecare formula:

- Who is this person?
- What are the person's eating patterns?
- What foods are culturally familiar?
- How is dementing disease affecting the person's nutritional status?
- What behaviors associated with eating need to be noted?
- Has the family been consulted about personal idiosyncrasies?

The following factors are considered:

- the level of nutritional risk
- strategies for lowering that risk, including providing suitable energy/protein requirements; creating a personalized meal plan; modifying the texture of foods served; ordering a therapeutic diet; offering assistance with eating and determining the level of assistance; providing prosthetic dishes and utensils; and making changes to the overall Daily Care Plan

FIGURE 12-10

- caregiving approaches, and suggestions for change
- frequency of review needed

Once the person's nutritional patterns and nutritional risk level have been established, the team is in a position to begin designing the prosthesis for nutrition, the Nutritional Care Plan:

- *Energy requirements*

  First, the energy/protein requirement is determined. Does this person require extra protein or supplements due to daily patterns of activity? Is the person too distracted, anxious, or confused to access all the food needed for good health? Is special monitoring therefore required? Does the family supplement regular meals with extra food? Is the person eating other residents' meals? Is the person hoarding food from special-occasion meals? (See Energy Expenditures, Fig. 12-3 p. 227)

- *Personal meal planning*

  Once these questions are reviewed, a personal meal plan can be developed. This requires staff to determine the person's optimal times for meals, and how the 24-hour allotment of calories will be distributed throughout the person's day and evening. The following questions are considered:

  - Is this person someone who habitually eats a big morning meal, and then lighter meals during the rest of the day? Or is this someone who has never eaten breakfast, but habitually eats around lunchtime?

  - Is this a person who prefers several small meals offered throughout the waking period?

  - Are there favorite and hated foods?

  - Are there other food preferences to be considered and worked into the meal plan?

  - Does this person require modification of food textures because of poor dentition or dysphagia? This is a particularly contentious issue: all too often, because of staff or family concerns about choking, all of a person's meals may be pureed. This precaution can deprive people of much of the enjoyment

*A man seldom thinks
with more earnestness
of anything than he
does of his dinner.*

—SAMUEL JOHNSON

of eating; remember, texture, color, and presentation can often make up for losses of taste and smell. If a person has choked on toast, for example, soft pancakes or muffins can be safely substituted for toast, while still giving the person the pleasure of different food textures. If a person has choked on an apple (or had difficulty eating one), other, softer fruit such as pears, berries, or melon can be substituted.

Please note! These ideas are not just "frills"! Rather, they are creative therapeutic strategies which will enhance a person's nutritional intake. Once again: families are often willing to help provide special foods if they understand the meal plan the staff is attempting to implement.

- *Therapeutic diets*
Therapeutic diets can create eating problems. Such diets are sometimes required by people with dementia because of concurrent medical problems. However, most people with dementia are relatively physically healthy. Gentlecare recommends that each special therapeutic diet order be scrutinized very carefully by the interdisciplinary team. Many such orders are simply carryovers from another period in a person's life, and the conditions that prompted the diet may have changed in the interim.

- *Assistance with eating*
The majority of people with dementing illness need no help with eating, and in fact should be encouraged to eat independently if possible, in order to improve nutritional status. Better nutrition would prevent weight loss, resist infections and skin breakdown, and provide dietary fiber to combat chronic constipation problems.

The team needs to determine what, if any, level of assistance the person needs to be able to eat adequately. The following questions must be answered:

— If food is presented appropriately, can the person manage eating independently?

— Does the person respond better if food is presented one item at a time?

— Does the person need help initially only? Can he then follow through on his own?

— Does the person need periodic "kick-starts" to combat apraxia?

— If so, what type of prompt works best—verbal, physical, or mimed?

— Does the prompting need to be sporadic only, or given fairly regularly throughout the meal?

— Does the person need total feeding assistance?

— Does the person need a liquid meal in a cup?

— Can the person feed himself if bowls, or spoons, or wet cloths under the plate, or other adaptive equipment is used?

— Can the person eat independently if offered finger foods rather than foods requiring the use of utensils? (See Gentle-care Finger Foods, Fig. 12.11 p. 242)

I ONCE WORKED IN A HOSPITAL *where every meal was scraped into a bowl, mixed with cold milk, and served as a lukewarm porridge regardless of the people's ability to chew or swallow.*

Remember: half the world eats exquisite foods with fingers only! As well, children—operating at developmental levels not unlike those of people with dementia—are not expected to manipulate complicated utensils.

• *Prosthetic dishes and utensils*

To compensate for physical or cognitive deficits, offer appropriate utensils:

— utensils with non-slip, built-up grips

— metal spoons—never the plastic variety

— plates with lips

— non-slip mats or wet cloths under plates

— colored glasses to provide visual contrast

A number of rehabilitative services offer prosthetic dishes and utensils that can help people maintain independence while eating; catalogues are available on request. However, much of

GENTLECARE FINGER FOODS

PROTEIN SOURCES
Cubes/slices of cheese

Cheese balls

Chicken nuggets

Strips of cooked meat or chicken

Fish sticks/sausage rolls/meat tarts

Hard-cooked eggs (halved)

Small meat balls

Crisp bacon

Sandwiches (egg, meat, chicken,
    peanut butter, tuna, etc.)

Grilled cheese sandwiches

Crackers with cheese, peanut butter

SWEETS
Doughnuts, doughnut holes

Cookies

Squares, brownies

Cupcakes, muffins

Biscuits with jam or jelly

Granola bars, yogurt bars

Ice cream, frozen yogurt cones

Popsicles, fruit juice bars

BREADS, ETC.
Toast fingers/cinnamon toast

Melba toast

Bread sticks

Pretzels/potato chips

Toasted English muffins

Lemon/banana/fruit bread

Cinnamon buns/rolls

Digestive biscuits

Pancakes

Arrowroots/social tea biscuits

VEGETABLES & FRUITS
Florets of broccoli, cauliflower

Mushrooms

Zucchini

Cucumber

Dill pickles

Cherry tomatoes

Home fries (warm)

French fries

Green or yellow beans

Carrot/celery sticks

Cubes of cooked turnip, potato

Apple or pear sections

Orange sections (no seeds)

Banana sections

Melon balls/wedges (no rind)

Strawberries/peaches

Seedless grapes

ETHNIC TREATS
Egg/spring rolls

Samosas/chapatis

Crepes/waffles

Almond/fortune cookies

Cornbread/polenta

Hors d'oeuvres

Scones

Cornish pasties

Fish and chips

Note: Some of these foods are not appropriate
    if the person has restrictions on diet due
    to medical problems. Most people with
    dementia can eat these items to improve
    nutritional status, prevent weight loss,
    resist infections, and provide dietary fiber.

FIGURE 12.11

this specialized equipment is very expensive, and often does not survive its first tour through the dishwasher. Gentlecare recommends that staff and families search through stores specializing in equipment for kitchens, children, and sports to find creative solutions to the need for adaptive equipment. Finding such items can also be made a special assignment for volunteers/families.

- *Physical positioning*

Physical positioning of both the person eating and the person assisting with some aspects of eating are critical for successful nutrition. The person who is eating should be positioned to be able to both see and reach food:

— If the person is eating in bed, raise the bed to an angle of at least 60°, and place firm pillows behind shoulders and neck. The person should be positioned in a slightly flexed position with chin down to close the airway.

— If the person is eating in a chair, the person's head, shoulders, and arms should easily clear the table top. Low chairs are a significant cause of decreased independent eating function because over time, they cause a person to lose arm function and then to give up trying to eat.

The person who is assisting with aspects of eating must be positioned so as to enhance the skills of the person who is eating.

If total assistance is required, the suggested position for assisting is on the dominant side of the person being helped; seated on a moveable stool that locks at the height of the person being assisted; and slightly ahead of, facing, and at approximately a 45° angle to the person being assisted. This position allows the person assisting to check swallowing and chewing activity, which can't be done if the helper is directly opposite the person being helped, or if the helper is working at a feeding table.

If only partial assistance is required, the suggested position for assisting is on the dominant side of the person being assisted; seated on a moveable stool that locks; and positioned at the side of the person being helped, with both people facing in the same direction. This position allows the person who is assisting to move utensils toward the mouth by guiding the hand of the person being helped. It also permits the person being assisted to mimic appropriate actions. The assisting person may only need to repeat or kick-start activity from time to time.

Before eating begins, remove all restraints that might impede breathing. Keep throat and chest area free of towels or cloths used to clean the person's mouth.

Be sure the person's head is supported and controlled. Eating is a flexion-patterned activity; avoid hyper-extension, as it opens the airway and may lead to the aspiration of food.

- *Techniques for assisting with eating*

If a person has trouble controlling liquids in the mouth, try using the following:
  — liquids in slush form
  — foods with a high water content
  — gelatinized liquids
  — pudding, sherbets, ice creams
  — popsicles
  — fruit ice cones
  — commercial frozen snack products

Give only small amounts of food with each swallow. Ensure that the food is cleared from the mouth before introducing more. Use small spoons to introduce foods. Do not use the edge of the spoon to clear food from the lips and chin, as the skin in this area may be very fragile. Do not use syringes for feeding, under any circumstances, for any reason.

- *Triggering strategies*

When total assistance with eating is required, the following triggering strategies can be very helpful.

1. To trigger mouth opening:
  — Touch both lips with a weighted spoon.
  — Give a sip of water.
  — Ask the person to open her mouth.

- Place your fingers on the sides of the lips, or apply light pressure on the chin.
- Do not try to force the jaws open.
- Mime the mouth opening.

These techniques will also often help to open a person's mouth if teeth are clenched on a utensil.

2. To trigger lips closing:
- Stroke the lips with a finger, spoon, or ice popsicle.
- Apply manual pressure, holding your forefinger just above the upper lip and your thumb under the bottom lip to purse the lips together.

3. To trigger tongue movement:
- Try icing the tongue.
- Place a cold spoon lightly on the tongue.
- With a tongue depressor, touch the tissue just behind the lower teeth; the tongue will "follow" the touch. DO NOT USE YOUR FINGERS!

4. To trigger saliva production:
- Try icing the tongue with a favorite popsicle.
- Try plain ice.
- Try sips of water.
- Try a salty or savory bit of food.

5. To trigger the swallowing reflex:
- Touch the person's chin or throat gently to stimulate the digrastic muscle.
- Give a sip of water. This will often help a person with Alzheimer's disease to understand that food is present in the mouth.
- If food is still in the mouth, offer an empty spoon to trigger swallowing.
- Try icing the sternal notch and rubbing the back of the neck with a washcloth.
- Lightly pinch the pharynx.
- Bring food into the person's visual range.
- Offer the person the food to see and smell (for example, a piece of fruit or bread).

I think the feeding is the hardest part right now, it really is. . . . I'm sorry to say my patience runs out and sometimes I just give up. . . . I wish, I wish I could understand why she doesn't open her mouth and why she doesn't swallow.

—MARY,
A CAREGIVER

— Use hot or cold liquids rather than tepid ones.

— Remember that textured foods stimulate swallowing more than liquid or pureed foods do.

Use discretion if there is a history of choking. Remember that many choking incidents are more likely to have resulted from poor assisting techniques and/or poor positioning than from an actual inability to swallow.

- *Encouraging eating*
  - Use special treats to trigger the eating response. Serve them with water as an appetizer before meals.

    Gentlecare Appetite Trigger foods—small pancakes with jam; crisp bacon strips; curly, seasoned potato fries; potato chips; cheese cubes; fruit juice popsicles; and salty crackers.

  - If a person is disinterested in traditional main course foods (meat, potatoes, and vegetables) or simply finds eating a full-course meal too complex or exhausting, try the following.

    Gentlecare Meal Substitutes—(Families are often willing to help with provision of special foods.)

    –buttered zucchini and date loaf with cheese, hard or cream variety;

    –banana bread with peanut butter and a glass of milk;

    –Milk, tapioca, or rice or bread pudding, fortified with eggs, milk powder, and/or a nutritional supplement, and garnished with jelly, jam, or syrup;

    –baked custard with caramel sauce, maple syrup, or jam;

    –tarts filled with vegetable/egg/milk mixture and/or meat or fish;

    –chicken or fish strips, nuggets, or sticks, with bread and butter and pickles;

    –thick cream soups with meat, fish, and vegetables;

    –chunky soups (split pea soup with ham, fish chowder, corn chowder) with crackers;

    –baked beans with hamburger or wieners, cut up, with chili sauce added;

–a dish of fruit with raisin or cinnamon bread and butter and a chunk of cheese;

–assorted sandwich plate (egg salad, minced ham, chicken salad, peanut butter and jam, etc.);

–poached or scrambled eggs on toast;

–creamed peas on toast, creamed salmon on toast, with pickle or chili sauce;

–banana split with ice cream or frozen yogurt, custard sauce, and canned or fresh fruit;

–plain yogurt garnished with cut-up fruit and oatmeal/ peanut butter/chocolate chip cookies or digestive biscuits or bread with peanut butter;

–hot cereal (oatmeal, cornmeal, cream of wheat) fortified with wheat germ and/or bran and a nutritional supplement, with whole milk and brown sugar;

–milk shakes made with whole milk, skim milk powder, and fruit (banana, etc.); and

–applesauce with warm gingerbread and a glass of milk or a scoop of ice cream.

Remember: only foods that have been mixed with a liquid (saliva, water, juice, etc.) can be tasted!

Some of these suggestions are obviously not applicable if there are therapeutic diet restrictions on fat, sodium, or total calories. Most contain a combination of protein, fat, and carbohydrates that is approximately equivalent to a moderate serving of the traditional first course of a meal.

• *Food textures*

— Experiment with a variety of food textures, from soft to chopped, minced, pureed, or liquid. Remember that a person may be able to manage several different levels of food texture, depending on the food itself, the assistance available, the temperature, etc. For example, a person may require assistance with porridge, but be able to eat finger foods like pancakes or muffins independently.

— Encourage the person assisting to identify the food being presented after two or three bites.

— Give clear, simple, concrete instructions: "Open your mouth," rather than "Open up"; or "Clear the food out of your mouth," rather than "Swallow it."

— Use the disease dysfunction of *hyperorality* (the apparent need for oral stimulation) to assist with eating: place a small sample of the food near the mouth.

— Check for visual field neglect (inability to visually perceive objects on one side, usually the left) and place items of food within the person's visual range. Be sure items are not outside the reduced peripheral field of vision.

— Offer ongoing encouragement. Eating is so very difficult that any support aids the person in the effort to cope.

— Avoid feeding tables. They infantalize older people and place staff so that they are not in a position to correctly assist with feeding and cannot monitor swallowing. People with dementia often need to mime the action of staff, so they lose ability to eat in direct proportion to inappropriate feeding technique.

I RECALL WATCHING AN ELDERLY LADY *being escorted to her place in a very large, noisy dining room. Her dinner tray was placed in front of her, with the dish covers in place. She sat quietly with her hands in her lap. Once or twice staff members urged her to eat. One offered her a sip of juice. Toward the end of the meal another staff member paused and said, "I guess you're not hungry tonight." She then removed the tray and scraped the food into the garbage pail.*

Without appropriate knowledge, the staff members missed the problem of apraxia—the woman's inability to initiate eating—with devastating consequences.

THE GENTLECARE 24-HOUR NUTRITION CLOCK

Gentlecare has developed a program of strategic metabolic boosts that enhance performance, avoid nutritional low points, and prevent catastrophic behavior (see Sundown Syndrome, p. 234). This strategy spreads out the daily nutritional allotment over the 24-hour cycle with a possible 10-point nutritional boosts.

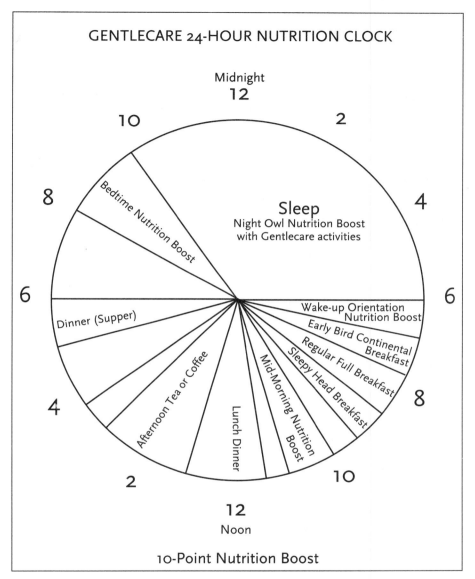

GENTLECARE 24-HOUR NUTRITION CLOCK

Midnight

Sleep
Night Owl Nutrition Boost
with Gentlecare activities

Bedtime Nutrition Boost

Dinner (Supper)

Afternoon Tea or Coffee

Lunch Dinner

Mid-Morning Nutrition Boost

Sleepy Head Breakfast

Regular Full Breakfast

Early Bird Continental Breakfast

Wake-up Orientation Nutrition Boost

Noon

10-Point Nutrition Boost

FIGURE 12-12

1. Wake-up and orientation nutrition boost;
2. Early Bird continental breakfast;
3. Regular full breakfast;
4. Sleepy Head breakfast;
5. Mid-morning nutrition boost;
6. Lunch (or dinner);
7. Afternoon Tea (or mid-afternoon nutrition boost);
8. Dinner (or supper);

9. Bedtime nutrition boost; and

10. Night Owl nutrition boost.

This system does not encourage people to eat whatever they want, whenever they want, or as much as they want—it should not be confused with the dreadful notion of "grazing." Grazing is the practice of putting food out in an informal setting and letting people make choices, and it is particularly inappropriate for the cognitively impaired. Dementia sufferers lack the judgement and are often too medically fragile to be able to manage buffet-style eating. Remember that each individual has a specific care plan that indicates nutritional needs and preferences. For example, a person who likes to sleep in would enjoy the Sleepy Head breakfast rather than the Early Bird continental. Staff members and family can both assist the person to access the appropriate meal or nutritional boost.

Each individual care plan indicates which of the 10 possible nutritional boosts are served to the person with dementia. Some individuals may receive four or five meals, while others get six or seven, depending on their needs.

Under this system, meals tend to be smaller and mid-morning, afternoon, bedtime, and nighttime nutrition boosts tend to be more substantial and nutritious. To assist digestion, sugar, and empty calories are avoided; caffeine and meat is avoided for the Night Owl nutrition boost.

In selecting foods for elderly people, be aware that caffeine is not well tolerated. It is found in beverages such as coffee, tea, cocoa, soft drinks, candies with milk chocolate or dark chocolate, prescription drugs like Soma Compound or Darvon Compound, nonprescription drugs such as weight control aids, alertness tablets, analgesics/pain relief, diuretics, and cold/allergy remedies. All of these contain sufficient caffeine to warrant their avoidance.

We prepare a 24-hour clock for each individual based on his/her nutritional needs. Once individual nutrition plans are developed, people can be grouped with others as early birds, sleepy heads, or regulars to facilitate dining times.

Review of the Plan

Once the nutrition care plan has been developed, it must be reviewed by caregivers who know the person well—professionals and family members. Before the plan is finalized, everyone must agree that it is a good one, especially if they are to take part in carrying out the recommendations.

Once the plan is agreed upon, everyone is expected to comply with it. Any concerns or proposals for change must be reviewed by the team, agreed upon, and documented so that everyone involved is aware that a change has been made.

The team also needs to agree on how often the nutritional care plan is to be reviewed. Dementing illnesses are diseases in transition; the nutritional care plan must change as often as is necessary to address alterations in a person's needs.

Documentation of the Plan

The final step in the creation of the nutrition care plan is the documentation of the decisions made in a form that is convenient to read and accessible to all. The vital information in the plan should be easily communicated to anyone who reads it: family members, care staff, volunteers, and any support staff who may assist with the person on occasion.

Step 5: Staff Compliance Check

Gentlecare elicits the assistance of all staff, family members, and volunteers who help people with dementia at mealtimes throughout the course of the day. It is critically important that each of those people understands the importance of nutrition and the specific nutritional requirements of each individual. Caregivers must also understand the difference between nutritional requirements for energy and performance and nutritional preferences. Nutrition is serious business!

People experiencing Alzheimer's disease are at risk of developing protein-energy malnutrition because of a combination of poor food intake and increased energy requirements. Therefore, institutions need to develop a monitoring system that ensures all staff and care providers

Gentlecare seeks to make mealtimes as pleasant, relaxing, and complete a social experience as possible for each individual— regardless of his degree of dysfunction.

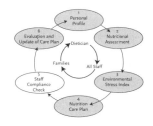

FIGURE 12-13

Bless the food that
comes to me,
With those who share
and serve it.
And if there be a
good dessert,
Oh grace me to
deserve it.

—A.F. BROWN

FIGURE 12-14

10 GENTLECARE SUGGESTIONS FOR GOOD NUTRITIONAL CARE

1. Educate your staff to see eating as a principal therapy, and train them to assist with eating skillfully and gently.

2. Make food and meal-related activities part of the program for each day.

3. Find creative solutions to difficulties with handling food. Provide appropriate seating, utensils, and dishes to make independent eating easier. Try finger foods.

4. Provide appropriate, attractive eating areas.

5. Be flexible and creative about mealtimes, menus, food textures.

6. Provide frequent, high-energy nutritional boosts.

7. Reduce noise levels/stress.

8. Watch for possible dehydration problems.

9. Keep nutritional assessments and care plans up-to-date for each individual in your care.

10. Set up ongoing communication between departments to promote Gentlecare strategies and problem solve quickly.

understand and comply with each individual's nutritional care plan. Staff compliance with respect to the nutrition care plan must be checked one week after implementation of the plan, or as appropriate to the level of risk and/or rate of change in status for each individual.

Step 6: Evaluation and Update of the Nutrition Care Plan

The final step in the nutritional management cycle is the evaluation and update of the nutrition care plan. This critical phase ensures that the foods provided each person with dementia match the individual's special and changing needs. The care plan is revised at intervals determined by the person's nutritional/health status or risk; considered at least biannually at a multi-disciplinary care conference. The continuing repetition of the nutritional management cycle is a guarantee of quality in overall management of care.

FIGURE 12-15

13

The Magic of
Gentlecare Meals

"It's the loveliest time of my day!"

In Gentlecare, we regard meals as the feature of the day rather than as a mere function. Mealtimes can be powerful therapeutic intervals, not just pit stops. In addition, the energy derived from eating and drinking can be used to smooth over the difficult times, and give people the means to perform the very difficult task of living with cognitive impairment. Eating therefore becomes a critical point on the ascending and reinforcing spiral of daily activity of Gentlecare.

The following sections illustrate how the basic core activity of eating can be integrated with other, higher levels of activity: necessary activities, essential activities, and activities that give meaning to life. These four levels of activity can be integrated into each of the five core activities of toileting, grooming, bathing, dressing or eating. In this way, any Activity of Daily Living (ADL) can become the basis of Gentlecare's Powerpoint activity program, and provide opportunities to promote exercise, enhance communication and socialization, promote dignity and respect, and support achievement, however basic the level.

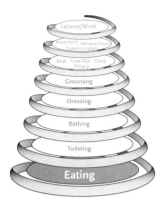

FIGURE 13-1

Eating: Core Activity

Eating is one of the essential Activities of Daily Living (ADL). The goal of Gentlecare programming is to use the ADLs as the basis for therapy instead of separating therapy or a single ADL as an individual entity. Food should be provided not three times a day, but as many times as necessary, to accommodate smaller appetites and minimize dips in energy. Mini-meals should be provided upon awakening both in the morning and during the night, and at bedtime. These meals should be offered in quiet locations, often in conjunction with family visits or quiet activities.

Associated Necessary Activities Related to Eating:

In order to maximize the value of eating, rest periods are a necessary activity both before and after mealtimes. Rest activities should take place away from dining areas, and should incorporate music, fresh air, reading aloud, playing of family tapes, and/or wrapping in blankets to help reduce stress. Small, intimate dining spaces enhance privacy and improve eating function. Nutrition boosts like bedtime snacks and early morning wake-up treats enhance rest and sleep.

Associated Essential Activities Related to Eating

People should be walked to and from meals—preferably in the open air. Sometimes people can be danced to their meals. Marching works well, too!

Seating arrangements should use regular chairs and should encourage interaction. Buddy relationships (bonding with another person) should be encouraged. Avoid feeding tables. Often, residents can be introduced to a buddy, encouraged to look for each other and remind one another of mealtimes, walk to the dining room together, and sit together at a table.

Involve family in meals whenever possible—not to "feed" their loved ones, but simply to share a meal with them. Build family events such as birthdays and anniversaries into special meals. Talk about fam-

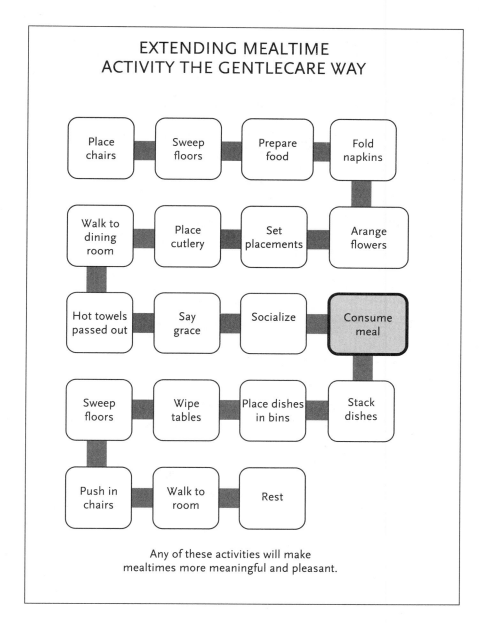

EXTENDING MEALTIME ACTIVITY THE GENTLECARE WAY

Place chairs → Sweep floors → Prepare food → Fold napkins

Walk to dining room → Place cutlery → Set placements → Arange flowers

Hot towels passed out → Say grace → Socialize → Consume meal

Sweep floors → Wipe tables → Place dishes in bins → Stack dishes

Push in chairs → Walk to room → Rest

Any of these activities will make
mealtimes more meaningful and pleasant.

FIGURE 13-2

ily, meal preparations, favorite foods, food costs, and food products. And watch your language at mealtimes: avoid such terms as "feeders" and "feeds".

Staff should sit on stools and not hover over people with dementia. Offer hot towels before and after meals. Massage shoulders while putting on clothing protectors or aprons. Avoid calling them "bibs".

Associated Meaningful Activities Related to Eating

All special events should be integrated with food: food discussion, food preparation, table setting, and flower arrangements. Activities can be tied into meals by providing opportunities for serving and clearing up, and translating those activities into work. Recipes can be discussed to sharpen interest in food. Filling the dining area with familiar food aromas has the same effect.

Meals should follow old rituals and customs, and be made special. Here's a true-life story told by Sandy Telford of the Deltaview Habilitation Centre:

Use color to influence eating patterns. Warm, mid range colors like red, peach, yellow make food look better and people hungrier. Cool colors like blue and gray have the opposite effect.

"IT WAS CORN SEASON IN B.C., *so we decided to serve corn on the cob in our Gentlecare unit. It was a great hit! Over 50 percent of our people just loved it. Even people who usually have to be fed, or who had not held food in their hands for long periods of time, eagerly ate the ear of corn. Some sucked on the end of the cob, others had corn and butter all over their faces, and one gentleman ate four cobs. Everyone had a glorious time.*"

The staff of Deltaview expanded the simple act of eating into a social and therapeutic event. They achieved dramatically different results than they would have if they had simply served corn niblets as a vegetable. Powerpoint programming, using corn on the cob, took people with dementing illness back to a time in life when corn season had been a joy for them. People were encouraged to recount their memories of corn feasts and were placed in a position of power: of remembering. The feelings of comfort, happiness, and competency in former life-roles directly translated into improvements in people's levels of functioning. This is a perfect example of the ascending and reinforcing spiral of activity in action.

Here's another illuminating example of how the presentation of food can enhance people's functioning in their total life context:

I VISITED A HUGE TOTAL CARE *treatment ward several years ago and watched as staff brought more than 100 people into a large dining room. Every person was in a wheelchair, geriatric chair, or bed.*

Every person in the room was served a tray of food, and without exception every person was either assisted to eat, or totally fed by staff. At the end of the meal, staff members returned everyone to their rooms.

The next morning I arrived before the breakfast hour, and was surprised to see people making their way independently to the dining room. Some were walking with the aid of canes or walkers; others were pushing wheelchairs in front of them as support, while still others pedaled their wheelchairs along with their feet. Long before serving time, many people were in their places.

Then I noticed that staff members were cooking pancakes and bacon at the side of the dining room. Wednesday morning was pancake morning! The buzz of conversation in the room was louder and more joyful than it had been the previous night at dinner. Many, many people were feeding themselves independently, using spoons and fingers, admittedly, but eating without assistance. People were talking one to another, passing food around the table, asking for syrup, and most significantly, asking for seconds! Very few staff members were involved in feeding activity. As I passed one old gentleman who had been morose the evening before, he looked up at me and grinned. "Good grits!" he said.

Armies march on
their stomachs.

—NAPOLEON
BONAPARTE

Staff members throughout health care services have witnessed similar transformations. When food looks like food, tastes like food, smells like food, and reminds people of former pleasurable times in life, eating becomes a pleasure rather than a chore. People's level of competence increases, and less staff intervention at mealtimes is required. When food is served in odd-shaped containers, with lids that can't be opened, on trays, and is managed by staff members, cognitively impaired people will not recognize the activity as eating. Consequently, if they are to eat, someone will have to feed them. Eating then becomes an onerous task to be completed (with the help of staff) as quickly as possible, rather than part of an ascending and reinforcing spiral of spontaneous and independent activities.

If we know this to be true, why do we persist in following systems of food preparation and presentation that result in accelerated dysfunc-

*The stomach supports
the heart, not the
heart the stomach.*

—OLD ENGLISH
PROVERB

*I phoned a special care
unit to ask if I might
visit. The charge nurse
said, "Sure, come and
visit us. We're making
pancakes and
peaches!"*

tion, increased staff intervention, massive waste, and higher costs? There is no good answer to that, but fortunately, more and more facilities are moving to a more flexible, normalized system of meal preparation and presentation to meet the challenge of dealing with dementia.

Many facilities are moving to buffet-style service, which allows people to make food choices, and possibly to serve some items to other diners or help in the layout and clean-up of food items on the buffet.

Other units are successfully using salad, dessert, or beverage carts, often incorporating residents as servers assisted by staff members. Several years ago I visited a unit in the Penticton Retirement Centre in Penticton, B.C., Canada. The dinner was being served from a mobile cart by the cook and assistants, complete with chef's hats. The chef went from table to table serving food, discussing choices, presenting various dishes for inspection. The level of participation, enjoyment, and discussion was just amazing. It is hard not to compare this experience with the long, noisy staff line-ups to collect trays, while people wait patiently at tables with their hands folded. Over and over again, experience has shown that it is not more expensive or time-consuming to offer meals in more creative ways. The more normalized the activity, the greater the payoff in terms of interaction, increased functioning, and better nutrition.

There is plenty of evidence to support the notion that when cognitively impaired people are comfortable, in control of their situations to the degree possible, satisfied, and provided with a home-like dining situation, they derive more benefit from their food. Indeed, this is true for any elderly person! Such a therapeutic nutritional experience occurs when staff members are empowered to work in interdisciplinary teams; when effective diagnostic and behavioral analyses are routinely carried out; and when family members are included in problem-solving.

Creative innovations to care can be successfully introduced when staff are informed and supported, and when they are encouraged to work in partnership with families.

PART FIVE

DESIGN FOR LIVING

GENTLECARE
The Prosthetic Life Care System for People with Dementia

UNDERSTANDING ALZHEIMER'S DISEASE

ASSESSMENT IN DEMENTIA CARE

A NEW APPROACH TO PROGRAMS

NUTRITION IN DEMENTIA CARE

DESIGN FOR LIVING

PEOPLE AND THEIR IMPACT ON CARE

14

Homematch

We shape our buildings,
and then they shape us.
—Winston Churchill

Home is where the heart is. Home is a magic word. In each of our memories there is a special place that we regard as home. It may be the place where we grew up. It may be the first home we lived in when we were married, or the place where we raised our children. It may even be a new location at the end of a busy lifetime. Home, in fact, may not be a building at all, but rather a place, treasured possessions, or a feeling of comfort and ownership.

I have been thinking a great deal about the notion of home and what it means to me. For me, home is the beautiful old stone house I lived in for the first 20 years of my life. I recently visited it for the first time in many years, and felt the rush of memories: my parents, my friends, my wedding. Each stone and tree held a story that I felt impelled to relate to my traveling companion!

Home is also the first home that my husband and I lived in. How could I forget the wallpapering experience? Developing our first garden? Or the place where we raised our son? For the last 20 years, though, I have lived in a big old house on Canada's west coast. Surely, this is home! This is where my family lives, where my dogs are, my plants, my books, all the significant memories of my adult life.

And yet, due to the nature of my work, I live much of my life in hotels. Are they my homes too? I can only say that the way I organize the hotel room is very important to me. Before I even think about working or answering telephone messages, I must unpack my bags, place my pictures and books just so, arrange my tea-making utensils and all my safety equipment, place some flowers in view, and organize my pillows. Then and only then, with this illusion of home around me, am I ready to take on the world.

If this is my experience, could the importance of home affect others in a similar way? Could the place they live in be an important factor in the way they view life?

Hospitals used to be the places one visited in a medical emergency, to recover from disease, or to have some dysfunction repaired. Despite feeling unwell or frightened, there was always a mystique about hospitals—the stuff of life-and-death TV dramas. There is always a sort of magic or fascination attached to a brief visit to hospital. And we always knew we would be going home again soon.

However, hospitals have now assumed functions other than the treatment of acute illness. Together with a variety of care facilities, hospitals have become places where some people stay for a very long time. In fact, many people—elders especially—live out their lives in these essentially institutional buildings, which have become their home. Within the complex organization known as a health care facility, elderly people now must attempt to find their room, their bed, their bathroom, their bouquet of flowers. For people experiencing dementing illness, this is a virtually impossible undertaking.

Hospitals are essentially designed as places where health care personnel work. The complex medical, institutional, and technological nature of that work inevitably results in settings that are counter-therapeutic for residents who must, instead, use the facility for daily living.

Recognizing the need to modify this workplace setting so that residents can feel at home, long-term care facilities have for some time now attempted to create a residential character by using home-like furniture and decorating styles. Unfortunately, many such efforts do not

You are a King by your own fireside, as much as any monarch in his throne.

—CERVANTES, *DON QUIXOTE*

Typical views from the living space of older people who reside in health care facilities.

Ask yourself this question: "If I stepped out of my room into these corridors would I know where I was, or where to go to spend the rest of my day?"

Example of attempts to develop a residential ambiance in the living space of older people within institutions.

A typical living room and bedroom in the home of an older person.

extend beyond front lobbies. They are often only window dressings—a marketing strategy rather than a sustained effort to create a domestic setting that people can control. For the most part, health care facilities for elderly people are places where residents know they should stay out of the way and be as inconspicuous as possible.

I have worked in a facility where a huge chain is placed across the dining room whenever meals are not being served so the room can be cleaned and remain tidy for the next meal. Such practices raise the question: When was the last time you were prevented from entering the dining room and food preparation area in your home by a chain? How would it make you feel to be excluded from an important part of your home? Would you feel in control of your life? Or would you feel like an intruder in someone else's space?

This is the dilemma facing elderly people when they live in health care facilities: how much like home is home? Only recently have there been serious efforts to assess the damage inflicted on people, especially elderly, cognitively impaired people, by the typical health care environment.

The negative effects of noise, glare, confusion, and rush are becoming matters of great concern to health care planners—and at the same time, the notion of the positive potential of the environment as a therapeutic force has everyone excited. What if, by changing the places where demented people live, we can change their behavior? For example, what if we move the television out of the main dining room (as a large psychiatric hospital did recently) and as a result, people stop yelling? What if we change the current practice of bathing people by undressing them, draping them in a sheet, and wheeling them on a chair lift through crowded corridors to a room that looks like a car wash, and instead help them undress in a room that looks and feels like a bathroom? What if we find that they then actually enjoy their bath time?

An example of removal of a door to a bathroom and replacement by a curtain.

What if we design bedrooms for elderly people that feel like regular bedrooms instead of hospital rooms? Might they then be more comfortable, content, compliant?

The possibilities of supportive environments are endless; they are limited only by our imaginations and creativity. For the most part, they are feasible and affordable. Putting a picture of a toilet on a bathroom door, taking off the bathroom door and replacing it with a curtain, improving the lighting between bedroom and bathroom—these approaches certainly cost less than using drugs or restraints to control an old gentleman who is searching for a bathroom, or worse still, devising his own toilet alternative.

Environmental adaptation does not cure dementing illnesses, but until a medical cure is available, developing people-friendly facilities goes a long way toward empowering cognitively impaired people. If we begin shaping buildings that people can enjoy living in, perhaps we can truly help people live through the devastation of dementia with some degree of comfort and dignity.

Let's examine the design principles that inform current building practices in health care. Space is typically allocated in descending order of priority:

- reception/administration
- nursing station/medication/records
- kitchen/food services
- dining room
- activity/dayroom areas
- rehabilitation/treatment areas
- patient rooms/bathrooms
- bathing areas
- cleaning/storage/utilities
- indoor/outdoor movement areas

Typical large surveillance station

This environment is designed with a view to providing health services as quickly and effectively as possible. Safety, cleanliness, infection control, and surveillance are the operative words. The large, centrally located nursing station is perhaps the best example of inappropriate and archaic design, one that informs the culture of a facility. None of us has any area in our homes that remotely resembles this design feature. Such an arrangement of space and equipment speaks loudly of hospital, not home. Nursing stations are focal points in a hospital because staff are located behind them. Staff are people's major support system: most people depend on staff members to monitor their health, give them instructions, and liaise with their physicians. Staff control discharges, money, meals, bath times, cigarettes, and contact with families.

When people suffer from cognitive impairment, this kind of control becomes a life issue. If a person has no area of independence, he must keep his support system in view at all times; without these key individuals to feed, dress, toilet, and communicate, only the black pit of dementia exists. How better to keep one's support system within reach than to sit in a convenient row of chairs placed in front of the nursing station? Across the barrier, one can keep help in sight at all times— even speak to someone once in a while, or be spoken to as staff members move back and forth behind the counter.

Meanwhile, behind the barriers, staff members are absorbed in the tasks of charting, telephoning, and discussing health status. The exhausting effort of talking to cognitively impaired people, trying to get them involved, dealing with the needs of families, or working on relationships with fellow employees—those challenges can be put aside in favor of the comforting routine of paperwork.

And so the architectural barrier, the nursing station, begins to shape the way we work and the way residents live. Professional caregivers become abstract managers of paper and things, and cognitively impaired people become voyeurs and supplicants, waiting patiently for that one magic moment of contact when someone happens to emerge from behind the counter.

When I ask architects why they build these "air traffic control centers," as I call them, they cite the need to meet numerous technical requirements: a need for staff to have an unlimited view, for surveillance of large numbers of people; a need to protect confidentiality; security;

and prevention of unacceptable resident access to computers, telephones, etc. However, everyone agrees that quality dementia care happens when staff mingle with residents. And we are all aware that sitting in a glass control center is an outdated practice. What facility has staff members available to sit and do surveillance anymore?

Most people would agree that security and confidentiality can best be achieved by the provision of an enclosed, out-of-sight room. Small, well-designed communication rooms where staff members can carry out essential phoning or charting activity, in relative calm, are beginning to replace traditional nursing stations. Not surprisingly, when staff can work in privacy, residents begin to use more appropriate living spaces, indoors and outdoors, abandoning the line of chairs in the corridor.

A new order of priority in long-term care facility design is beginning to emerge:

- resident room/bathroom
- activity areas
- social/dining areas
- bathrooms
- indoor/outdoor movement areas
- communication room for use by multi-disciplinary team
- kitchen/food services
- rehabilitation services
- cleaning/storage
- administration/reception

An example of a well-designed communications room.

This new emphasis views design from the perspective of the person who lives in the space rather than as a workspace for staff. It attempts to address the reality that many older people no longer simply pass through health care facilities, but rather live out their lives within them. There is an effort underway to capture the spirit and comfort of "home" as a means of combating the destructive interaction of dementia and institutionalization.

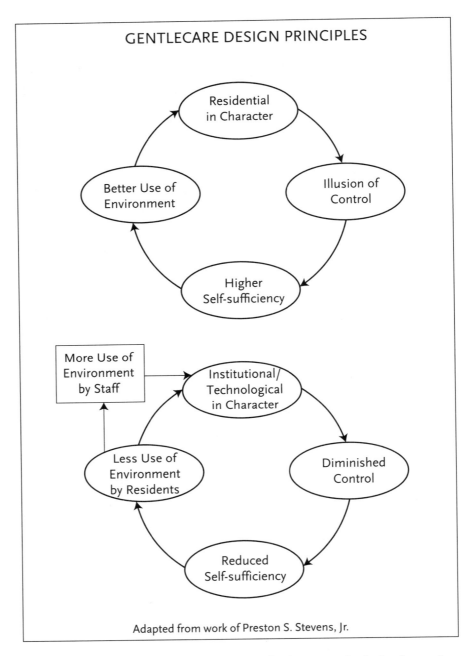

GENTLECARE DESIGN PRINCIPLES

Residential
in Character

Illusion of
Control

Higher
Self-sufficiency

Better Use of
Environment

More Use of
Environment
by Staff

Institutional/
Technological
in Character

Diminished
Control

Reduced
Self-sufficiency

Less Use of
Environment
by Residents

Adapted from work of Preston S. Stevens, Jr.

FIGURE 14-1

As we begin to assess the potential for harm or for help that exists
within environments, some basic principles emerge:

- Design should be sensitive to the needs of the users. Elderly
  people appear to be best served when they are in a home-like
  environment.

- Design should reflect the type of building being planned, as well as who will occupy the building. What will this building be used for?
- Design for social organization. Does this building permit or discourage social interaction?
- Design should respect the individuality of people, especially older people. No one design fits all.
- Design should take into account the effects of the disease process on the people who will use the building.
- Aging is a multi-dimensional process. Design should take into account the functional ability of each individual resident in terms of biology, psychology, and social reactions.
- Design for aging people must reflect sensory changes, especially auditory and visual changes.
- Design features should stress wellness, not illness.
- The scale of the building should not be overwhelming, but rather should be designed as manageable space for older people.

In the Gentlecare system, the physical environment is one of three critical elements (People, Programs, and Physical Space) that together make up the prosthetic program for people with dementia. Often, the physical space of Gentlecare is one element that people attempt to implement—because it seems easier, more concrete, quicker, and cheaper. But design of a prosthetic physical environment goes far beyond the installation of colored toilet seats or the use of non-glare wax.

The following design criteria (adapted from the work of Preston S. Stevens, Jr.) are fundamental to building the Gentlecare environmental prosthesis:

- The more residential the character of a building, and the more it resembles home, the more comfortable the person living there will be.
- The higher the comfort level within the building, the more people will feel in control of the spatial situations in which they find themselves.
- The greater the illusion of control people have, the more functional

they will be. One's level of self-sufficiency increases proportion-
ately to the sense one has of control over one's destiny.

- The more intact a person's level of functioning, the better the
chances of them making use of the environment.
- Finally, the more we live in and use an environment, the more we
will shape it into our personal version of home or residence.

Unfortunately, in the design of most health care facilities, the exact
reverse of this process is the norm. As Figure 14.x indicates, typical
health care facilities are institutional in nature, highly technological,
and designed for work efficiency and staff use. Residents who live in
such facilities feel uncomfortable and experience no sense of control.
Residents are heard to say: "Is this my bed?"; "Can I sit here?"; and "Is
it okay if I go out?"

As a result of their perception that they are interlopers in an institutional setting, they are reluctant to assert their abilities. They are afraid
to look after themselves, explore their environment, or make unilateral
decisions. As they become more helpless, they make less and less use
of the facility's space; typically, they sit for long periods in corridors, in
dayrooms, or in their bedrooms. The phenomenon of alienation from
the environment holds true for family members, as well.

Since people make little use of living space within the facility, staff
members begin to use it as work space. Corridors become filled with
laundry, housekeeping materials, medication carts, and storage boxes.
Areas are blocked off for dining only, or cleaning, or charting. Residents are moved to the periphery of the space. The physical environment becomes more and more institutional in nature: more and more
technology is put in place such as public address systems, alarmed
doors, wander-guards, even special sensors attached to people to alert
staff when they move about. As time schedules, routines, and staffing
patterns lock into place, they create a circle of influence that tightens
and tightens, choking off any home-like ambiance of the structure and
defining its use.

The feeling of place is a
power within us.

—JAMES REANEY

A TOUCHING THING HAPPENED *in a facility recently. I was working with a very imposing looking gentleman who was a stranger to the facility, as I was. We were approached by an elderly lady who said, "Are you the government man?" My associate acknowledged this by saying, "Yes, I do work for the government." "Do you have a ticket, then?" she asked. "A ticket?" "Yes, I want to go out to that concert in the park," she said.*

Tragically, residents often refuse to eat because they are afraid that they cannot pay the bills in the fancy restaurant. Or they are afraid they are in the way. Or they think the chair, the room, or the garden, belongs to someone else. All these perceptions, engendered by the environment, contribute to iatrogenic illness. By focusing on changing the physical environment, the Gentlecare system attempts to engage the remnants of personal power behind the disease in an effort to make cognitively impaired elders feel more comfortable and in control of their lives.

A DIRECTOR OF NURSING SERVICES *called me to say they had recently moved their cognitively impaired residents to a quiet area of the facility where they could move about indoors and in the garden if they wished. The staff had no budget to decorate or remodel the area in any special way, but they thought they would take this first step. She said, "Moyra, we simply couldn't believe it! Overnight we noticed changes in people's ability to eat, and groom, toilet, and dress themselves. They seemed so much happier and content. We can hardly wait to begin to make some real changes."*

15

Designed to Heal

In the fifth century B.C., Hippocrates, the father of medicine, was said to have taught his students outdoors, under a tree. The aesculapiums (the ancient temples of healing) were places to treat both body and soul. Greek patients were soothed by massage, mud baths, and herbal teas. Their minds were stimulated and healed with poetry, music, and drama.

Just as surely as architecture can dehumanize an environment, it can also help to humanize it. Since the major group in most health care facilities consists of elderly people, it is important to reflect on the human needs of these users of the system, and to design facilities accordingly.

Design Implications Due to Changes in Health Status

Research has shown that as people age, five specific spheres of function are affected: vision, perception, sensory integration, motor ability, and cognition. Gentlecare addresses the design implications of each of these functional changes.

Vision

The richest of the human senses, vision provides us with a wealth of information that has a decisive influence on our reactions, our ability to concentrate, our efficiency, and our general sense of well-being or fatigue. For many people, the first overt sign of aging is *presbyopia* (difficulty with near vision resulting from a loss of elasticity in the lens of the eye). People experience an extreme sensitivity to glare. Changes in levels, or perceived changes in levels of flooring due to colors or patterns, can result in falls. Reduced visual acuity means lighting levels must be augmented and colors chosen carefully.

When poor lighting combines with colors, patterns and texture—especially in crowded areas—the stage is set for elderly people to have problems. As a person's ability to distinguish varying levels of light intensity (as given off by color in patterned flooring, for example) the pattern gives the illusion of a step. As the elderly person responds to this perception, they lose their balance and fall. At the same time a lack of color or more significantly, a lack of a figure/ground contrast, can give older people the impression of being in a "whiteout". They have an unpleasant feeling of uncertain footing or an absence of solid footing which is very uncomfortable. Often they stop walking and remain in bed or in a chair in order to compensate.

Floor patterns appear as holes or steps to cognitively impaired people.

GENTLECARE Practice Tip

Gentlecare suggests staff members work for a few hours wearing very dark sunglasses, while at the same time assessing the effect this has on their functioning levels.

This quickly leads to loss of function. Many new buildings are decorated in popular colors of pink, peach, or beige with no contrast or grounding features to assist older people to move about comfortably.

It is generally agreed that elderly people (especially those with changes to brain tissue) require at least three times as much light as younger people in the same environment. Gentlecare recommends the use of natural light or incandescent light. Floor and table lamps can be bolted in place like those in motels, and track lighting can be used to provide illumination for specific tasks. Strong contrasts in light should

Glare, color, texture, and confusion all affect a person's ability to move comfortably.

be avoided: for instance, a dark bedroom should not connect to a brightly lit bathroom, nor should a bright corridor lead into a darkened room. Do not follow the common practice of dimming lights to reduce anxiety and agitation. Such a practice has the effect of putting elderly people into a blackout, and of course, then they do not move around. All these changes make it difficult to read and interpret the environment correctly.

Perception

As people age, and particularly if they suffer from cognitive impairment, the parietal lobe of the brain is affected. The ability to manage one's body in space and to perceive and understand environmental stimulation is impaired. Environmental design can either support failing spatial perception or further undermine it. Avoid at all costs the use of sconces which produce a dangerous pattern of light and dark that disorients older people, causing falls and fractures.

Pattern, juxtaposition of colors, and differences in light/dark contrast all affect the elderly person's ability to move safely and use space effectively. Every effort should be made to choose flooring without any pattern, and in warm mid-range colors. Carpeting should be constructed with a tight weave and a short strand length; smooth floor coverings should be slightly cushioned and have a non-glare matte finish. Glare is every bit as toxic for a perceptually impaired person as are rush, noise, and confusion. Avoid the currently popular use of dark borders in corridors. Such borders force older people to leap over perceived gaps in the carpeting, causing falls.

Parietal lobe damage also impairs a person's ability to correctly identify objects and locations. Identical corridors, bedrooms, or doors make it difficult for elderly people to distinguish their own room from those of others. Gentlecare recommends the use of good wayfinding cues, in both picture

CHANGES IN PERCEPTION

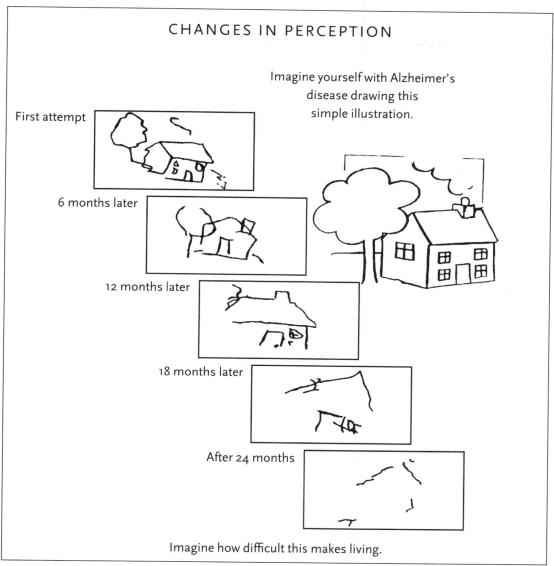

Imagine yourself with Alzheimer's disease drawing this simple illustration.

First attempt

6 months later

12 months later

18 months later

After 24 months

Imagine how difficult this makes living.

FIGURE 15-1

and word form. Familiar objects that break up the length of corridors give important sensory clues to cognitively impaired elderly people. As the brain ages (and all of our brains are aging!) our ability to perceive, identify, and integrate sensory stimulation (shapes, colors, textures, figure/ground definition, depth perception, and sounds) is impaired. A dark color may be perceived as a hole or drop-off; shiny floors may become lakes or skating rinks; and ordinary sounds can become oppressive and frightening. Most importantly, sensory integration is slowed down. Thus, elderly people who are rushed or in crowds cannot decipher stimulation quickly enough to be able to react appropriately, and are thus at risk for falls. They may also be frightened and anxious, due to misinterpretation.

Motor Function

As people age, muscular/skeletal difficulties occur. As a result, balance is impaired and reaction time is slowed. The ability to lift one's feet and manoeuver is compromised. Patterns, textures, colors, glare, rush, noise, crowds—all these combine to cause elderly people difficulties in mobility and functioning.

Elderly people lose muscle strength, and this is exacerbated by the fact that they often just sit for long hours. It becomes harder for them to move through large spaces, down long corridors, and around huge outdoor spaces. Muscle contractures, joint fusion, pain, and edema combine to prevent the older person from moving freely and making full use of the living environment and outdoor spaces. Designers must take this into account, arranging for smaller spaces, easier access, and safer footing.

Alzheimer's disease affects gait patterns and possibly leads to falls.

Cognition

As dementing illness destroys memory and memory-processing ability, the critical life function of learning is lost. A person with Alzheimer's disease cannot process new information. Thus a new location, new people, new procedures, and unfamiliar routines make life terribly challenging and difficult for a person with a dementing illness. People with dementia cannot remember directions; they cannot follow directions, or problem-solve their way out of strange places. They cannot differentiate their room from that of another person, especially if the doors are identical. They cannot find access doors, or even ask for appropriate information. If they do receive useful information, they forget it before they can use it.

People with dementia lose the ability to reason. Thus they cannot understand why they must bathe, or why we use a mechanical lift to assist with bathing. They cannot understand why they must sit in a certain location, or why they cannot lie down on a bed just because it happens to be assigned to someone else. They do not understand that messages conveyed over public address systems into their "home" do not apply to them, but rather are messages for other people. The ability to use one's mind to problem-solve one's way through a frightening and challenging environment slowly diminishes.

So how can we make a better match between our health care environment and persons' special needs? How can we make institutions feel like home? How can we achieve Homematch to limit the effects of illness and support residual function?

Critical Elements of the Prosthetic Environment

Safety and Security

People with dementia live out their lives in the physical space provided by the health care system. Because of the massive damage these people have suffered to memory, reasoning, and the judgement centers of the brain, the area in which they live must be secure and free from significant risk.

People with dementia do not understand why they are being asked to stay in a strange place, and many desperately try to leave—they want to find their home and family and attend to their responsibilities. In health care we give this behavior all manner of euphemistic titles: exterior wanderers, elopers, exit seeking behavior, etc. The hard fact is that the person doesn't feel at home and tries to leave to find his real home.

Thus perimeters of buildings need to be secured. Once this basic safeguard is in place, staff time is freed up to comfort and support the people with dementia, rather than being devoted to enforcement of building exit rules. The widespread reluctance to provide secure perimeters stems from troubling images of locked areas, ghettos, restraints, and prisons. However, if buildings housing elderly people with dementia are not secured, eventually physical and chemical restraint measures will be used to confine these vulnerable people to specified locations.

GENTLECARE DESIGN PRINCIPLES

The Gentlecare system develops living environments based on the following essential elements:

Safety and Security

People with dementia lack cognition, reason, and judgment. Their environment must have safe perimeters and their accommodations must be reasonably free from risk. Security measures must be as non-invasive as possible. Sound alarms should be avoided.

Access and Mobility

Due to confusion and disorientation, access must be clearly defined and lead the person into the appropriate areas. Good access should exist indoors and outdoors. Freedom of movement is critical to good dementia care. Walkways should be inviting, clear of obstacles, and lead the person to where they want to go, or to interesting objects.

Function and Activity

Prosthetic environments exist to be used by the people who live there. Opportunity for engagement, interaction, and meaningful activities should be non-intrusive and not distract from the home-like atmosphere.

Individual Control Privacy Comfort Sociality

People with dementia should be regarded as guests. The environment exists for their enjoyment and use. The physical space should be designed to invite or direct social contact, give comfort, and respect privacy.

Flexibility Choices Change Participation Decision-making

Dementia is a disease in progress. It involves a widely differing group of people. The environment should be designed to accommodate changing needs. The perception that this is the resident's home governs all activity.

FIGURE 15-2

It is sometimes helpful to compare our attitudes toward secure perimeters around children's daycare facilities, and our feelings about secure perimeters in long-term care facilities. No one would consider placing a child in a program that allowed unrestricted access to busy streets, yet we do not speak of daycare centers as locked units or prisons. It is expected that organizations caring for children arrange for their safety and security. In fact, so ingrained is the practice of securing buildings that house children that we scarcely ever discuss the issue.

Yet every day, health care personnel fight and struggle to keep people with dementia from leaving buildings and wandering into dangerous traffic. Staff members spend endless time running after escaping people and attempting to persuade them to come back. They notify family members, often in the middle of the night, that their loved ones have eloped.

Dutch doors, murals, or distracting objects can often keep people with dementia from exiting doors.

New technology is regularly introduced into health care institutions: alarms, buzzers, and sensors are designed to warn staff that a resident is exiting without permission. The pandemonium that results when the alarms go off drives everyone crazy, residents and staff members alike. Alarms are rapidly becoming the new frontier of restraint. There has to be a better way—and there is.

Many health care facilities use silent key-pad operated locks to provide security at exit doors. The code for the lock is posted, so staff, visitors, and cognitively alert residents can exit and enter at will. Frequently these doors are

Contrast the difference between these two gardens. One is inviting, while the other could be perceived as a prison.

camouflaged by painting the door the same color as the adjoining walls, or by placing a distracting or interesting object in the corridor several feet before the door to engage the attention of residents.

Fences are the best method of securing the exterior perimeters of a facility. If the fence is attractive, natural, and interesting, it can serve as an effective security measure. If the fence is oppressive, bare, and ugly, it may encourage the idea of escape.

People with dementia face other risks as well. In an effort to promote safety, health care institutions often eliminate every conceivable risk factor. As a result, special care units or dementia areas become unstimulating places where people with Alzheimer's disease wander meaninglessly through empty rooms and up and down bare corridors, or walk back and forth on cement walkways outdoors. Plants are forbidden because they might be poisonous. Pictures and curtains are eliminated because people might tear them down. Personal possessions are ruled out because someone might steal them. All small objects are eliminated, because someone might swallow them. Such attitudes subject elderly people to safe but empty, meaningless lives. We would never dream of raising children in such a bleak atmosphere, even though they are certainly capable of all the risk behaviors just mentioned.

Of course it is very important to ensure that elderly people with dementia do not come to any harm. However, experience has shown that the more residential the environment, the more appropriate the behavior of the person with dementia will be. Units that abound with beautiful, interesting, meaningful objects that offer support and comfort to people with dementia bring out the best of their remaining function. Natural plants create a familiar atmosphere that evokes a former life, and provide hours of meaningful work. (See Figures 15.3 and 15.4 for a list of toxic and non-toxic plants to be included in indoor and garden design.) Gentlecare avoids artificial plants, which confuse people with dementia and do not give the same joy as natural ones.

The world begins to exist when the individual discovers it.

—CARL JUNG

Collections of interesting objects in baskets, trunks, dressers, desks, or hutches provide points of interest and endless hours of rummaging opportunities. Families are urged to supply generic objects or replicas of their loved ones' treasured possessions; thus, if another person becomes attracted to a particular object, it can be replaced without problems or recriminations.

Safety is important, but it must be kept in perspective and not be allowed to overshadow the opportunity for a meaningful life experience.

Access, Mobility, and Wayfinding

Freedom of movement is critical to quality dementia care. Walkways should provide appropriate orientation and support to help people navigate their living space successfully. Both indoor and outdoor walking spaces should be provided.

It is preferable that pathways lead people to interesting locations or objects. Seating areas where people can rest are desirable along walking routes.

People experiencing dementia suffer from disorientation. Written

Life panels, often designed by family members, help people find their rooms, and give them reassurance, ownership, and a sense of being someone special.

signs have limited usefulness for them, so Gentlecare recommends using comforting objects to identify significant spaces or personal rooms: for example, artwork, quilts, grandfather clocks, desks, bookshelves, or large plants.

This doesn't look like any typewriter I've ever used!

Sometimes small treasures can be found.

Rummaging is a great way to pass the time.

Hat collections are fun and intriguing.

Moving furniture about is a wonderful means of exercise.

Furniture arrangements and interesting objects draw people with dementia into an area without the need for staff intervention. Gentlecare refers to such environmental arrangements as *non-human caregivers,* because of the pleasure and comfort they give and the fact that caregivers do not need to be involved.

WALK THROUGH AREAS *in a facility or home as if you were contemplating living in the space. Check out the rooms for their livability. Are areas clearly defined? Are interesting objects in view? Is the area comfortable, inviting, personalized?*

Small social areas filled with beautiful objects give pleasure all day.

Design access to the outdoors. Gentlecare recommends providing interesting objects that lead or entice people to the outdoors. Combinations of grass and asphalt provide safe walking experiences. Wooden decks are useful and comfortable.

Function and Activity

Celebrate people's competency and remaining function. Provide environmental opportunities for people with dementia to do normal, everyday activities. Try to achieve activity, interaction, and conversation through environmental design. To compensate for sensory deficits:

- Place interesting, fragrant, textured, visually attractive objects within reach of residents. Objects that are placed out of reach

A familiar clothesline outside a door invites an elderly person to participate in activity.

These objects cannot be seen or used.

do not exist in the minds of people with dementia, and therefore serve only as token attempts to create interesting environments. Furthermore, if sensory-stimulating materials are locked away in cupboards or placed in a special room, access to stimulating activities becomes dependent on staff involvement.

- Personalize.
- Individualize.
- Normalize.

Familiar activities like visiting or reading the newspaper are encouraged.

- Stress continuity with the past and former good times through the use of life panels, powerful 8 x 10 pictures of the person at significant times in life—for instance, at his wedding.
- Leave objects in plain sight.
- Display treasure chests, chests of drawers, baskets full of objects.
- Place antique objects in view.
- Use giant fabric flowers, birds, or animals.
- Enlarge photos, especially old familiar ones.
- Place real plants in the room that can be smelled, picked, and watered.
  - Arrange tasks that are in progress to entice people to become involved. Any activity is a good one if the person enjoys it, and no one else is harmed.
  - Place tools and work supplies in clear view.
  - Provide rummage opportunities.
  - Design privacy opportunities— small, quiet hide-outs where elderly people can go for rest, serenity, and time alone.

Beautiful spaces help alleviate the effects of dementia.

- Design quiet and active areas.
- Design redundant cueing in the environment. Use any method to make information available (verbal, visual, olfactory, tactile). Use pictures, smells, textures. Arrange for whiffs of familiar odors: coffee, toast, bacon, ginger, baking (yeast), lemon, tomato, cedar chips, cut evergreens, lavender, flowers, and perfume.
- Design shady areas protected from the wind. Include rain shelters. Elderly people do not enjoy direct sunlight or drafts. Use arbors, trellises, umbrellas, canopies, and large open, lighted gazebos. People with dementia will not enter small dark gazebo structures.
- Avoid a design that is park-like, or emulates a large public garden, sports ground, or playground ambiance. People with dementia will be afraid to enter such an area because the scale is overwhelming.
- Use a variety of leading points of interest to entice people into the garden and around the walking areas.
- Design walking pathways with edges flush to the ground. Pathways do not need to go in circles. It does help, however, if the path eventually leads people back to the door of the building.
- Highlight existing trees and plant additional ones for shade.
- Hang bird feeders, bird houses, and hanging plants from tree branches.
- Include piles of wood and places to pile wood as part of the garden.
- Install clotheslines against walls so people will not walk into them, with small tables for a clothes basket. Circular clotheslines work well, too.
- Set aside an area of dirt piles, shovels, wheelbarrows, etc.
- Install a dog house.

Arabian tents provide inexpensive and effective shady areas.

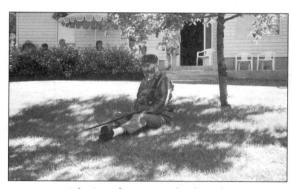

The joy of one's own backyard.

People with dementia have a tendency to direct their gaze downward. Objects above shoulder level are rarely enjoyed by them and are therefore of no therapeutic value.

Contrast the ambiance of the institutional emptiness of the space above with the backyard comfort and relaxation depicted below.

Raised flower beds give extra comfort to elderly people as they are easily accessed.

- Bird baths are magic! Surround them with seating to create a viewing area.
- Avoid fountains, pools, fish, and lily ponds unless you want to be on a toileting routine! People with dementia are both frightened and fascinated by water. They will wade in pools and will need to go to the bathroom if they hear or see water.
- Set up a mail box.
- Create a back porch effect, with shelter and appropriate furniture.
- Use large flowers like daisies and sunflowers, and fast-growing dramatic vegetables like zucchini and tomatoes.
- Cover fences with flowering vines and grapevines.
- Include some grass in the garden, and provide a push lawn mower.
- Some facilities use old cars, motor bikes, or bicycles for a work activity such as washing, polishing, or tire kicking.
- Set up a habitat for rabbits, ducks, etc.
  - Consider placing an old-fashioned pump in the garden.
  - Camouflage fences with shrubbery. Gentlecare uses flowering vines like clematis, Virginia creeper, or wisteria, and vegetables like beans, spaghetti squash, or sweet peas. Place clotheslines against fences or woodpiles. These designs distract from the feeling of being walled in.
  - Outdoor gardens should resemble and feel like an older person's backyard.
  - Balance safety with independence. Keep outdoor areas simple and normal.

- Often families or community organizations will sponsor and help care for a garden area. Make sure they understand the concept of a working garden in dementia care, so they don't create a park or a formal garden.

Low walls give a feeling of privacy in a busy dining room.

Individual Control, Privacy, Comfort, and Sociality

- Focus on wellness.
- Get rid of illness-oriented spaces and other reminders of incapacity in the environment. Place nursing stations, medicine carts, dirty linen, housekeeping supplies, supply cupboards, and items for storage in less prominent areas of the facility. Camouflage the doors leading to such service areas, and make the areas as inconspicuous as possible. Avoid medication carts in dining rooms; distribute medication before or after meals, not during them.
- Avoid large open spaces. Design small interesting environments at the entrance to the yard, the dining room, or any large open space so as to entice people into that space on their own.
- Design to a residential, not institutional, scale that is manageable from the perspective of the person with dementia.

The use of a Dutch door reduces the amount of space and stimuli that a person must cope with, thus reducing anxiety and exhaustion. This is the most benign form of environmental restraint.

- Arrange the life of the person with dementia around family clusters of four to six people, to minimize overwhelming interactions. In Gentlecare, for instance, meals are offered in small family-sized groups, rather than being presented to large numbers of people in large noisy dining rooms.
- Focus on individuality and personal ownership: each person should have some private space.

Flexibility: Choices and Change

- Use music and TV selectively.
- Place TVs in separate viewing rooms so residents can choose to be in a quiet room if they prefer. Avoid using TV or stereo as background or as a babysitting activity: people with dementia cannot remove themselves, protest, or make adjustments in volume. TVs should not be watched by staff members while they are on duty.
- Design space for family and volunteer use. Make them feel welcome.
- Abandon notions of neatness and order. If they are to achieve activity and interaction, dementia units should have the appearance and ambiance of a well-used home.
- Avoid shiny, polished, patterned surfaces.
- Patterns that have fine details tend to confuse, and should be avoided. Floral patterns that contrast strongly with the background color can increase confusion. Abstract patterns and stripes can appear to move or shimmer. Still-life patterns can be confused with reality, and should be avoided. The same is true of decorative murals or life-size drawings.
- Avoid the use of mirrors and glass blocks.

Space should be developed for use by volunteers and family members.

- Reduce noise pollution, especially in dining rooms. Avoid the use of background music, and turn off public address systems; ask staff to speak softly to one another; reduce the clamor by using rubber-tired equipment; hang acoustical wall hangings; install acoustic ceilings; install wall carpeting to waist height; divide large space with partitions; minimize random noise; and develop a policy of zero tolerance for noise in your facility.
- Color schemes should use warm, mid-range hues; cool colors appear washed out and sharp color contrasts can be uncomfortable.
- Chairs and sofas should have high seats, sturdy arms, and no support pillars between the front legs. Their functional purpose

should be clear. Bean bag chairs are actually a restraint and should not be used, since an older person cannot get out of them easily.

- Furniture should have rounded edges and an uncomplicated design.
- Use tall, sturdy plants for aesthetic interest and to change the atmosphere in a room.
- Boost illumination, especially in the afternoons and evenings. Use portable or standing lights for tasks, and to give a sense of comfort and security. Bolt lamps to tables.
- Illuminate changes in floor surfaces. Avoid sharp color contrasts, confusing patterns, and fine detail in flooring patterns.
- Use indirect and diffused lighting to reduce glare and shadows. Light levels should be consistent across all areas. Use warm white fluorescent light. Use more than one source of light. Illuminate entrances.
- Use cluster furniture arrangements to encourage socialization.
- Develop clear circulation pathways to promote security and competency.
- Use partitions to block the view of larger, potentially frightening spaces.
- Design "bus stops" or rest areas to provide opportunities to stop on the way to and from the dining room. Even a chair to lean on can help.
- Design bathroom facilities in close proximity to dining/activity rooms. Make them easily accessible and have them clearly identified.
- Check the functional relationship between the heights of dining chairs and table height. A person's arm should be able to clear the top of the table easily.

Contrast these two living spaces. One looks like a furniture storage area, while the other is filled with interesting things to do.

An example of a non-human caregiver . . . an inviting space.

- Arrange hutches and/or sideboards with familiar and interesting objects, pictures, and flowers. Create a mood or theme that reflects the natural lifestyle of elderly people.
- Keep corridors short or break them into sections by placing objects on one side of the corridor only, to facilitate movement.
- Design to a residential scale, rather than to a hotel or commercial scale.

To assess the perspective of the elderly person, lie on his bed to see what he sees.

- Avoid large waiting room spaces in front of the nursing station. Eliminate glass barriers, counters, or enclosures that separate staff from residents. Design to encourage staff/client relationships and interaction.
- Design bedrooms to permit a variety of bed locations.

- Design display panels at the entrance to people's bedrooms to enhance cueing and staff knowledge of residents.
- Focus display boards, picture groups, or furniture at the foot or the side of the bed so that the person in bed can see them. Avoid displays at the head of the bed. Sometimes photos can be more easily seen if they are placed on the ceiling or low down at the side of the bed.
- Design ledges of windows so that they are wide enough for plants, books, or other objects.
- Use small desks or work tables in rooms to encourage activity.

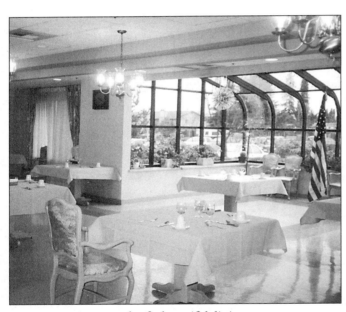

An example of a beautiful dining room.

- Dining rooms should be special places.
- Make dining rooms visually appealing and distinctive for older people. This should be a special room; places where people eat should be beautiful, quiet, and relaxing.
- Use square tables for four or round tables for six to encourage socialization and visual contact.

- Place tables at an angle to the wall rather than parallel to it so people can be seated or depart easily.
- Arrange small, intimate dining areas that remind people of home.
- Avoid large institutional spaces designed for dining activity only. They are noisy, crowded, and formidable for people with dementia. Use portable panels or half-walls to break up large dining spaces into quiet, manageable areas. Try using narrow planters mounted on wheels that lock as adjustable partitions. Furniture arrangements can also provide for the partition of space.
- Supervisory personnel should be conveniently stationed but discreet.
- Gentlecare recommends the use of the old-time family kitchen or family room that encourages not only dining activity but socialization and work.
- Use flexible seating arrangements so people have new dining partners at different mealtimes.
- Avoid the use of feeding tables. Such equipment infantilizes elders, causes difficulties in perception, promotes helplessness, diminishes functional ability, and can cause choking.

Bathrooms

- Bathrooms and bathing areas should be designed to protect privacy, dignity, and safety.
- Fixtures should be color-contrasted with

Contrast the atmosphere of family rooms or kitchens with the ambiance of a feeding table.

Clearly designate the room's function on the door of the bathroom. Avoid abstract designs.

Fixtures should be contrasted against the wall and floor of the bathroom for easier identification.

the walls and floor of the bathroom to make them easier to see and recognize.

- Cupboards for storage purposes should be provided in bathrooms. Rooms should be decorated with hanging plants (we use artificial ones in bathrooms), pictures, and beautiful objects. Include a towel warmer for comfort.

In general, reduce the amount of space and the number of stimuli elderly people must cope with. Anxiety and exhaustion can be significantly reduced if people are protected from over-stimulation. The most benign environmental restraint is the Dutch door; during monitored periods it allows residents to rest, and often to sleep.

Special Care Units have been criticized as serving merely to segregate troublesome dementia victims from other residents, but actually they should be the critical physical space of the prosthesis of care.

Plants: Toxic and Non-toxic

The use of living plants in a facility can make it much more homelike and functional; however, there are concerns about the use of some plants, which can be toxic if eaten. The following lists can be used as guidelines for unsafe and safe plants. Whatever you do, don't deny older people the joy of plants and gardens.

TOXIC PLANTS

The following plants are considered poisonous and possibly dangerous. They contain a wide variety of poisons, and symptoms may vary from a mild stomachache, skin rash, or swelling of the mouth and throat to involvement of the heart, kidneys, or other organs. A poison control center can provide specific information on these plants and others that may not be on this list but can be poisonous. *Many plants do not cause toxicity unless eaten in very large amounts.*

anemone	angel's trumpet (red sage)
apricot kernels	arrowhead
avocado (leaves)	azaleas
betel nut palm	bittersweet
buckeye	buttercups
caladium	calla lily
castor bean	cherries (wild and cultivated)
crocus, autumn	daffodil
daphne	delphinium
dieffenbachia (dumb cane)	devil's ivy
elderberry	elephant's ear
four o'clock	foxglove
holly berries	horse chestnut
horsetail reed	hyacinth
hydrangea	iris
ivy (Boston, English, and others)	jack-in-the-pulpit
jequirtity bean or pea	jerusalem cherry
jessamine (jasmine)	jimsonweed (thorn apple)
jonquil	laburnum
lantana camara	larkspur
laurel	lily-of-the-valley
lobelia	marijuana
mayapple	mistletoe
moonseed	monkshood
morning glory	mother-in-law plant
mushrooms	narcissus
nightshade	oleander
periwinkle	peyote (mescal)
philodendron	poinsettia
poison hemlock	poison ivy
poison oak	poppy
pokeweed	potato sprouts
ranunculus	rhododendron
rhubarb (leaves)	rosary pea
star-of-bethlehem	tobacco
tomato (except fruit)	tulip
wisteria	water hemlock
yew	

Do not further confuse elderly people with dementia by using artificial or silk plants.

FIGURE 15-3

NON-TOXIC PLANTS

The following plants are considered essentially safe and not poisonous. Symptoms from eating or handling these plants are unlikely, but any plant may cause an unexpected reaction in certain individuals.

african daisy	african palm
african violet	airplane plant
aluminum plant	aralia, false
araucaria	asparagus fern
aspidistra (cast iron plant)	aster
baby's tears	bachelor buttons
bamboo	begonia
birds' nest fern	bloodleaf plant
bougainvillea	camellia
Christmas cactus	chrysanthemum
coleus species	corn plant
crab apples	creeping charlie
creeping jenny (moneywort, lysima)	
croton species	croton (house variety)
dahlia	daisies
dandelions	dogwood
donkey tail	Easter lily
echeveria	eucalyptus (caution)
eugenia	fuchsia
gardenia	gloxinia
grape ivy	hibiscus
honeysuckle	hoya
impatiens	jade plant
kalanchoe	lily (day, Easter, or tiger)
lipstick plant	magnolia
marigold	monkey plant
Norfolk island pine	orchid
Oregon grape	pepperornia
petunia	piggy-back plant
prayer plant	purple passion
pyracantha	rose
rubber plant	salal
sansevieria	schefflera
spider plant	Swedish ivy
umbrella tree	violets
wandering Jew	wax plant
weeping fig	zebra plant

Any activity is a good one if the person enjoys it, and no one else is harmed.

FIGURE 15-4

Living space for people with dementia should be:

- normal
- home-like
- therapeutic
- non-technological
- prosthetic
- warm mid-range colors

They should avoid patterns that dominate or move, have comfortable objects and pictures, and be, in short, just like home.

FIGURE 15-5

PART SIX

PEOPLE AND THEIR IMPACT
ON CARE

16

People as Prosthesis

The world breaks everyone, and afterward
many are strong at the broken places. . . .
—Ernest Hemingway, *A Farewell to Arms*

In his lovely book *The Notebook,* Nicholas Sparks writes about Alzheimer's disease:

It is a barren disease, as empty and lifeless as a desert. It is a thief of
hearts and souls and memories.

In Gentlecare we have studied dementia in great detail, noting the destruction it creates in its victims. We have shared the horrors of the bleak reality that for many of these diseases there is no known cause, and therefore no cure.

In our search to discover how to help people live through the experience of dementing illness, Gentlecare introduces the paradigm of the prosthesis of care: three critical elements of support that provide families and others who care with a way of helping. These three elements are people, programs, and physical space.

Of the three, the people component is by far the most powerful. People are the therapy.

The world of the person suffering from dementing illness is populated by a variety of people. There are family members; there are many types of professional care providers; there are volunteers and important community service organizations. People in each of these categories have an impact for good or for harm on someone in the throes of dementing illness. People are important in any type of undertaking; but people *are* health care.

Dementia care, wherever it occurs, depends upon quality of service, flexibility, constant problem-solving, and innovation. Quality care is predicated on knowledge, skill acquisition, and ongoing training. It relies on respect, intuition, compassion, and dedication which, in turn, all depend on people.

Good dementia care relies on people working in complex interdependent relationships, giving of themselves, and putting out for other human beings in ways that are quite unheard of in any other relationship or service. Gentlecare believes that the people, lay or professional, who provide health care services to the victims of dementia are more important than the things that are used in the system or than the systems themselves.

Family Members as Carers

From the onset of Alzheimer's disease, the victim's family, and specifically the designated primary caregiver, is intrinsically bound up in the disease process.

Gentlecare regards the family as integral to dementia care, and works to support the family caregiver and sustain family involvement in the care of their relative to the very end of the process. In the course of the illness family members gradually assume responsibility for the person with dementing illness, answering questions, providing information and orientation, speaking on behalf of the person, and managing the person's grief as well as their own. Family life becomes consumed by the disease itself and by the burden of the care that must be taken on. Former roles as wife, mother, daughter, and friend are lost in a new, overwhelming job—caregiver.

This can be disconcerting not only for the family, but also for the person on the receiving end of the care. Without doubt, the sick person needs a caregiver, and yet there is something very sad about the loss of relationship that inevitably occurs when there is such dependency. The phenomenon is often referred to as role reversal, that is, adult children taking responsibility for their parents, or more frequently, a spouse caring for a life partner.

Family members often express their intolerable pain over the loss of interaction and connectedness with their sick family members. They express their grief over the loss of relationship: not having someone there for them, no longer being able to rely on a husband, being unable to confide in a mother. Alzheimer's disease makes these normal activities impossible. The people with dementia, too, often feel the loss of normal roles acutely, which accentuates their anxiety and sense of helplessness. We can hear this in frequently repeated remarks: "I can still do it" and "Don't tell me what to do!" More sadly, we hear it in their despair:

"One of the most difficult things for me is having a body in the house, but no one to talk to, to share news with...."

> "I can't do it. I can't handle it. I'm not asking you or begging you
> to fix me up so somehow I can but I've got to have some worth. I
> don't want to lose that too. I'm worth something—something
> other than this thing. But I don't have the wherewithal to do any-
> thing about it. I don't have any way to do it."

Once Alzheimer's disease strikes, the focus shifts from a normal relationship to new roles for both parties: those of "caregiver" and "care receiver." At the same time, family members are expected to assume incredible responsibilities, with little in the way of knowledge or specific skills; in effect, they become pseudo-professional care providers.

The person with Alzheimer's disease, on the other hand, is expected to fit into a new role: that of someone needing and receiving care. Yet we are often surprised when people don't accept that role graciously or willingly! Just at a time when these sick people are terrified and confused, they are asked to abandon former life roles and relationships in favor of a diminished existence controlled by others. As the disease worsens, there is less and less emphasis on normal life activities; the disease eclipses all life roles and functions.

Within the health care system, the family member who has Alzheimer's disease is often thought of in terms of illness, and the family caregiver is frequently assessed in terms of their role in dealing with the illness. In the process, it is sometimes forgotten that these two people have been husband and wife for perhaps 35 years. But when family members of Alzheimer's victims shift out of normal relationships and into new and unnatural roles as caregivers, do we lose a powerful therapeutic force? We all know extraordinary caregivers. Some family members go far beyond what most of us consider humanly possible to support and assist their loved ones. My mother was one of those.

And when I think about such caregivers, I am struck by the observation that their primary overriding focus is on the familial relationship rather than on their role as caregiver.

My mother, for example, learned all she could about the disease, and was very innovative in trying different approaches and strategies. But first and foremost, my father was her husband, and she did everything humanly possible to respect him in that capacity to the day of his death. When I listen to other such exceptional caregivers, I hear this repeated over and over:

People are the therapy.

> "Of course, I didn't know Dean while I was growing up, but when she got ill, I wanted to be the daughter she'd never had" (Joyce Wright, of her mother-in-law).

> "I plan to keep Wendy with me. She is, after all, my wife" (Tom Pope).

> "As long as I am able, I will be here for Andy. That's just my place in life" (Florence Renaud).

> "You won't ever leave me, will you?" "No, no...I won't ever leave you, George" (Helen Wilson).

Understanding The Dynamics of Family Caregiving

A person experiencing Alzheimer's disease typically lives at home with his family for an average of four years before professional help is sought, but we all know family caregiving can go on for much longer periods. The path of the caregiving experience only too often follows a steady decline into burnout.

At the time the disease is first identified, the family typically is thrown into a state of shock. Often the information is so horrific that there is a tendency to block out the whole issue: denial of the severity of a problem is a human and understandable way of protecting against intolerable pain. However, as the disease unfolds, the family must begin to make important decisions affecting the sick person—at the same time that they must provide increasingly difficult levels of care. They begin to experience anger and frustration over their inability to reverse the diagnosis, find appropriate help, or make the whole disease process simply disappear from their lives. The anger surrounding caregiving is very frightening. It may be displaced in many directions:

I don't like the role of caregiver.

—THE WIFE OF AN ALZHEIMER'S SUFFERER

- toward the medical community, which seems powerless to help;
- toward other family members, who may not be as involved as is deemed necessary;
- toward friends and neighbors, whose lives are untouched by disease; and/or
- toward the person with dementia, who is becoming more needy every day.

It is very important for family carers to understand that anger on the part of caregivers is appropriate! It is how we manage feelings of anger that challenges us

Such a diffuse and unfocused anger engenders a feeling of being out of control, and that emotional reaction is often misunderstood by the caregivers themselves, family, friends, and professional health care staff. All may consider the reaction to be dysfunctional.

It is very important for family carers to understand that anger on the part of caregivers is appropriate. Dementia is one of the ugliest diseases imaginable, and few of us who have felt its impact on our lives have not felt incredible rage. And rage can occur over and over again; it can lie in wait to sabotage one's emotional life at any point.

TOGETHERNESS

He used to be a part of me:
We shared in all.
He used to tell me what
he thought or wanted,
And I agreed, or argued for my way:

Result: a compromise. It worked!
We walked together and
chose a path we liked.
Then came dementia for him.
He became different —
mostly sad and lost —
And so was I.
We could not freely share;
We could not choose together;
we each were angry and
could not help each other.
Our world turned upside down.
Today it's tragic for us both.
He cannot make connections.
I feel alone;

he resents my helping him.
He cannot see, he cannot hear,
he cannot put his words together
He is adrift in a strange sea
And my little boat holds only me.

If we could only feel together
through this awful sickness,
It would help so much.
If I could only understand him
when he speaks;
If he could only know I want to help;
We'd both feel good again.
But no! Each day seems worse.
We cannot learn to work and
feel together

We fail and struggle hopelessly
in joint dementia.
Only one vague hope remains
Will there be part of me —
A bit of warmth and life and joy —
When he is gone?

— Gil Ludeman

I REMEMBER AN EXPERIENCE of long-delayed anger in my own life. Years after my father died, I was walking along a street and went into an antique shop to browse. I paused to look at an old mirror and was suddenly totally overcome by a rage so overwhelming that I ran out of the store and walked for blocks, trying to get my feelings under control. I remember feeling so angry that Dad was gone, furious that he wasn't here to share our favorite activity of antique hunting. It just wasn't fair. My anger manifested itself physiologically as well as emotionally—and most frightening of all, it was not under my control.

In our culture, anger is not a socially acceptable emotion. From childhood on, all of us, but most especially women, have learned to suppress feelings of anger, to express our rage in alternate ways. But anger not addressed is internalized, causing depression or dysfunctional behavior. Caregivers need to be reassured that anger must be expressed. It must come out. But it is important that we learn to focus our rage in appropriate ways.

People with dementia need families more than ever.

It is not appropriate to direct anger at ourselves. It is equally inappropriate to direct anger at the person with dementia who is totally vulnerable, unable either to understand or to change, and who can suffer terribly in an atmosphere of simmering anger. Sometimes anger can best be expressed through effective advocacy on behalf of our loved ones or for all persons suffering with dementia. Support groups, therapists, grief counselors, and sometimes friends also can help families to understand their anger. Most important of all, the factors causing anger must be changed. The life circumstances that cause us so much distress must be identified and modified. For example—

- if a family member does not seem to be doing an appropriate share of caregiving;
- if a longtime friend never comes by;
- if some part of the disease has not been explained thoroughly;

- if someone who isn't participating in the caring is critical of those who are;
- if the person with dementia does something we don't understand; or
- if the health care system does not seem to be providing appropriate services

then there is a requirement for analysis and resolution of the issue. Otherwise, the anger created will end by undermining your health and performance as a caregiver.

As family members attempt to steer their way through both the maze of dementia and the bureaucratic hurdles of the health care system, they can experience frustration more intense than they have ever felt in their lives. And much of this is due to sheer lack of knowledge. One of the persistent myths of Alzheimer's is that the less people know about the disease progress, the less frightened they will be. Gentlecare opposes this approach, believing that people are never as afraid of what they know as they are of what they do not know. Families need to understand what is to come, or they will never be able to make appropriate care happen.

ONE DAY I WAS CALLED *on the telephone by a very elderly lady who appeared to be in deep distress. She said to me with tears in her voice: "No matter what I do, he gets sicker and sicker every day. I cook his favorite meals. I dress him in his favorite clothes. But every day he gets sicker and sicker."*

I said, "But, my dear, that's the nature of the disease. Alzheimer's is a progressive disease, and you will not be able to alter the fact that your husband is losing abilities day by day."

Her response was, "I didn't know that. No one told me it was going to be like this." Then I said, "It's simply awful. But even though he is going to become less able to do things, there are still all kinds of things you can do that will make your lives more comfortable." And I shared with her some of the strategies we use in Gentlecare. In a much more cheerful and determined voice she said, "I'm going to try some of those things."

A few days later her son phoned me. "I don't know what you said to my mother, but you've saved her life!"

Now, nothing so spectacular had happened; but what I had been able to do was to give her the information and knowledge she needed in order to do the caregiving job more effectively. I was able to empower this already strong, dedicated woman to do her job more effectively.

The anger and frustration of the early stages of the disease give rise to debilitating anxiety and guilt as the family's control over the disease, and consequently over their lives, slowly fades. Not knowing what's happening, not knowing what to do, sensing changes in lifestyle that haven't been planned for or even discussed, watching the sick person slipping away—all these feelings contribute to an emotional paralysis.

Family caregivers feel helpless and disheartened. They question themselves and others, critical of a system they see as contributing to the impotence in which they are trapped. These thoughts lead inevitably to the trademark feeling of the family caregiver: guilt.

Guilt is one of the most malignant of all the kaleidoscope of feelings the family caregiver experiences. It is a heavy, unwarranted burden that saps the caregiver's spirit and steals energy. Arising from unresolved anxiety and helplessness, the expression of guilt appears more socially acceptable than the admission that one's life is being controlled by a relentless disease—and that circumstance makes one very angry.

Family members who may have cared for sick people for hours, days, months, and even years will claim to feel guilty if they take time for a bath; and our social and health care system reinforces this notion of culpability. It's not unusual for people to be urged to keep their sick family member at home rather than seek professional help, even at the expense of their own health. I can vividly recall my mother being counseled by a health professional team: "You've been married all these years. Surely your husband deserves to live at home with you!" Few caregivers can resist pressure of this type. It is often easier to continue an intolerable regime of care than it is to chance public censure.

It is hard to imagine that a family member would feel guilty or would be made to feel guilty if they were seeking medical assistance for

I'm for sure not a sick-a-bed that needs Meals on Wheels! No, come on! I mean, there are other people who need that, and they should get it.

—A PERSON WITH ALZHEIMER'S

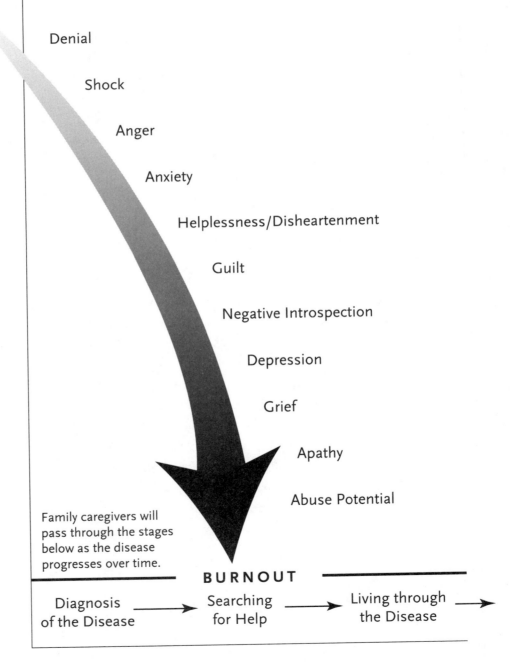

THE DYNAMICS OF FAMILY CAREGIVING

Denial

Shock

Anger

Anxiety

Helplessness/Disheartenment

Guilt

Negative Introspection

Depression

Grief

Apathy

Abuse Potential

Family caregivers will pass through the stages below as the disease progresses over time.

BURNOUT

Diagnosis of the Disease → Searching for Help → Living through the Disease →

THE PATH TO RECOVERY

Review of Life Choices

Stabilization

Healthy Grieving

Constructive Planning

Positive Introspection

Stagnation

→ Contemplation → Making Life Choices

FIGURE 16-1

a family member's cardiac disorder. However, the stigma of diseases of the mind prevails, and often profoundly informs behavior that affects people's lives. Guilt is a burden family caregivers don't need!

It is hard to be surrounded by the mini-deaths of progressive dementing illness and not feel oppressed and sad. Without support, caregivers can be overcome by negativity, anger, and helplessness. These negative feelings can lead to profound depression, which can last throughout the course of the disease and beyond.

Family caregivers are greatly at risk for clinical depression and rarely seek or receive treatment for this serious illness. Some research suggests that 40 to 60 percent of caregivers are clinically depressed. Depression not only makes caregiving intolerable for the person offering care, but it dramatically affects the functioning of the person with dementia. People with dementia are acutely aware of the feelings this disease engenders among others in their environment, and are unable to find respite from that oppressive knowledge and burden.

Overriding every other feeling, however, is the smouldering pain of grief. The grief that follows physical death is understood and accepted by our society. But grief associated with chronic illness is frequently ignored or misunderstood. Sometimes family caregivers will say, "I can't understand why I act the way I do; or why do I seem to be crying all the time; or why do I get so mad at him?" Rarely do they identify these emotional outbursts as emanating from prolonged, overwhelming grief.

Mourning someone who has not physically died, and who therefore falls outside the universally recognized rituals of mourning, places caregivers in an odd position: no flowers are sent; no sympathy cards arrive in the mail; no sympathy phone calls are received; and in fact, no one may call at all.

And yet death surrounds the caregiver. With dementia, unlike physical illness, the sick person is physically healthy for much of the duration of the disease process. What is grieved by the family is the death of the personality—the loss of the essential human being.

The grief associated with the small daily deaths or devastating changes (loss of skills, roles, dreams, and hopes) is often submerged in the overwhelming task of just coping with every day. Dementia care leaves little time for introspection. And the opportunity for an open examination and discussion of feelings rarely occurs, because the person with dementia is almost always close by.

So the grief of dementia is clandestine: grief is hidden, repressed, or changed to a more socially acceptable emotion like guilt. If caregivers admit to feeling bereaved, they are often reminded that the person with dementia is still alive. It is easier and more socially acceptable to be guilty than to grieve when you have lost a loved one to Alzheimer's disease.

Caregivers of people suffering from dementia are seldom considered to be bereaved prior to the actual physical death of their family member.

Society provides little opportunity to deal with the acute feelings of loss and grief that families feel throughout much of the process of dementing disease. Caregivers can't mourn decently while the person with dementia is still alive. Even within the family constellation, confusion can exist about mourning: often the spouse, as principal caregiver, is acutely aware of the extent of the disease, while other relatives see the person in social situations where functional deficits are concealed. But it is important to remember that grief neglected, grief ignored, grief scorned, or grief put on hold comes back to haunt us. Any time the pain and sorrow due to loss are not dealt with, the feelings will be manifested somewhere, some time.

Family members who acknowledge their grief and receive support and therapy, talk about a weight being lifted from their lives. They speak of renewed energy and a greater understanding of the actions of the sick person.

Help with anticipatory grieving is rarely discussed with families, nor is it readily available. Without such help, families continue down the slippery slope into a state of apathy. This classic feeling of helplessness is the inevitable outcome of chronic fatigue, sorrow, and isolation.

I have come to believe that abuse is a predictable outcome of the experience of caregiving, especially if that caregiving is carried out without appropriate respite, support, and therapy.

Lack of respite is the Achilles' heel of the family caregiver. Abuse

You are lucky . . . at least your husband is still alive. Mine died with a heart attack.

—WIDOW, TO AN
ALZHEIMER'S
CAREGIVER AT A
GRIEF SUPPORT
MEETING

Guilt is . . .

- never being able to say no
- never being able to satisfy the expectations of others
- never being able to satisfy yourself
- being angry in a nice way
- not feeling good about your best efforts
- being annoyed by others who expect you to be different, better
- stressful
- putting off making important decisions
- putting off taking action
- grief on hold, not examined, put aside
- expectations out of step with reality
- never being able to enjoy yourself
- feeling a failure
- feeling abused, used, left out
- narcissistic
- lonely
- ugly

Guilt uses all your energy and ruins your life.

FIGURE 16-2

occurs, it seems to me, in one of two ways: either the family caregiver sacrifices his or her health in an attempt to meet the needs of the person with dementia; or the caregiver goes beyond the breaking point and physically or psychologically abuses the person with dementia. Both types of abuse are systemic and pervasive in dementia care. Frequently the care giver is not aware of what is happening.

I REMEMBER BEING ASKED *to work with an elderly caregiver who had tied his wife to a tree in the backyard with a rope. When I asked him why he had done this, he said, "Moyra, I just can't keep up with her any more. I'm too old. She loves being outside, but I can't take her for walks any more."*

Abuse is an emotion-laden word these days, and most of us are reluctant to admit that caregivers, family or professional, would ever do such a thing. But abuse takes many forms: yelling, criticizing, isolating, restricting movement, leaving people alone, not supplying them with information, forcing them to eat, withholding food or drink, admonishing them, or making them feel responsible for some problem. All of these actions are just as damaging as the more commonly described physical types of abuse such as pushing, hitting, or neglecting.

We all need to become more sensitized to the potential for such action. We need to acknowledge that any one of us could react in a harmful way if we were physically and emotionally exhausted. We need to say to caregivers, family or professional: "Abuse is not OK, but it is understandable; and further, we will help you through this crisis."

Family caregivers who manage alone for years with no respite or support are greatly at risk. Professional caregivers who work with minimal resources are equally vulnerable. The potential for such problems needs to be brought out in the open, anticipated, and planned for, so that the well-being of neither caregivers nor care receivers is compromised.

Regardless of the order or severity of the feelings discussed, the outcome far too frequently is caregiver burnout. Burnout refers to a state of exhaustion, helplessness, and ill health that renders caregivers unable to care for themselves or anyone else. The Caregiver Burden Scale illustrates the typical decline in caregiver health over a five-year period (Fig. 7.7, p. 109).

The more we know about family caregivers, the more likely we are to be able to support them in their efforts to sustain the person with dementia.

I hope you understand when I say, I wish this would end!

— A CAREGIVER

I REMEMBER ONE EVENING, *working for a caregiver support group. As the family caregivers gathered in the room I became aware of a stifling burden of pain and loss pressing down on me. The room*

*Let us try to help the family caregiver
find their loved one behind the disease.*

was simply filled with sorrow. It seemed to me to be impossible to teach new ideas, or ask these caregivers to talk about their experiences. So I asked my colleague, who just happened to be a pianist, to play some music for us.

For several minutes he played "Memory" from Cats for us. As the music filled the room, the caregivers began to cry. I began to cry. And the terrible weight of pain began to lift and recede. Too often, the family caregivers just need permission to be human—to let go of responsibility, if even for a few minutes.

It is significant to note that most of the care for people with dementing illness is provided by elderly women. This fact should shape our efforts to assist caregivers in appropriate ways. For example, when we offer caregivers respite, what type of holiday or rest break do we have in mind? It's important to remember that older single women may not be used to traveling on their own, and may not have the money, clothes, or skills necessary to plan a vacation on their own. And older women are often perceived as half of a couple when they visit relatives or friends.

ONE OF MY CLIENTS, *while visiting relatives, was asked, "Where's Charley?" When she replied that she had left him in a wonderful respite bed in the hospital, they gasped in disbelief. "You left him where?"*

Data from an important study (Isenhart; reported in the *American Journal of Alzheimer Care and Related Disorders and Research,* October 1992) on the differences among family caregivers suggests that men and women offer care differently. In fact, people of different sexes may

DIFFERENCES IN KIN CAREGIVERS
OF PERSONS WITH DEMENTIA

Female Spouse Caregivers	Daughters and Daughters-in-law as Caregivers	Male Spouse Caregivers	Sons of Caregivers
Family orientation	Feel moral responsibility	High desire and commitment to relationship	Role confined to decision-making and financial assistance
Nurturing	Use parent-infant model of care	Take charge of care of ill person	Very low stress, depression, and burden
Extension of responsibilities	Keep parents at home for longer periods and at higher level of disability than is wise or appropriate	Motivated by positive forces	Use family and friends to help
May be saddled with care		Few guilt feelings	Use social services more effectively
May feel resentment	Fewer financial and emotional resources	Use assistance from other family members	
More depression	Higher divorce rates	Use social services	
More stress	Tend to refuse outside help	Can afford services	
Accept little or no help		Can identify problems, assess strengths and limitations	
Do not use social services	Low rate of use of social services	Less stress and depression	
Take more responsibility than reasonable	Feel guilty and overburdened	Action-oriented approach	
Under physical and emotional strain	Are stressed and depressed		
May conflict with other family members			
Become isolated			
Most in need of help			
Most difficult to reach		*"She deserves it."*	
		"She cared for me and the family."	
		"It's due her…"	
"No one else could handle him."			—Adapted from the *American Journal of Alzheimer Care and Related Disorders and Research*, October 1992
"I would feel so guilty."			
"This is my whole life…"			

FIGURE 16-3

even offer different types of care. The study further states that mid-life children have different approaches to the task of caregiving. What is significant is the variation in impact of the caregiving experience on personal health of men and women. Women caregivers clearly give more of themselves and become sicker in the process. Men, on the other hand, view dementia care as a job. They analyze the task, assemble resources effectively, and attack the job with an action-oriented approach. The Isenhart study suggests important insight that family caregivers can acquire to help them offer caregiving more effectively and protect their own health while doing so. Caregiving is clearly a risky business! The following is a summary of some of the factors to take into consideration when undertaking the job of caregiving or assisting someone else in doing so.

Alzheimer's disease affects all members of the family.

I have mentioned the fact that a majority of family caregiving is provided by women, and further, that men and women provide care differently. A significant factor in this difference appears to be the nature of the relationship between the giver and the receiver of care before the person became ill.

Today she couldn't tie her shoe. Can you imagine? She couldn't tie her shoe! What will be next?

If there is no pre-morbid history, as may be the case with in-laws, or if a dysfunctional relationship existed before caregiving began, then the challenging experience of caring for the dementia victim through the disease process will be even more difficult, if not impossible. A great deal depends on the personal health of the caregiver. Caregiving is exhausting, physically strenuous, and psychologically harrowing.

The organization of the living arrangements where care is to be provided is critical. If an aging parent with dementia is to be introduced into the family, consideration must be given to the displacement of other people, a loss of privacy, and the invasive nature of the disease it-self, to name only a few factors. Clearly, all members of the family must be willing to participate fully or the arrangement will be unsuccessful.

No matter what the living arrangement, it's important to remember that the person with dementia cannot change behavior, so adaptation must be the responsibility of family members. Not infrequently, several family members are involved in caring for an elderly parent, and this is not easy. If several people are involved, it's very important to decide on the primary caregiver. Then the whole family must support that person's decisions and efforts.

"Dad looks OK to me! We had a long talk about that fishing trip we took up north."

—A SON

If the person with dementia is to be maintained alone in his own home or in an apartment, arrangements are required for round-the-clock support. Often a live-in therapeutic companion can be helpful in this regard. The key to success, however, is stringent screening, thorough training, and supervision of employees.

Family Life Stressors Outside of Caregiving

Daily life goes on despite caregiving responsibilities. Interfamily conflict (whether between siblings, spouses, or children) can be devastating.

Caregivers are often faced with the additional task of buffering warring factions, or running interference for the person with dementia. This places an intolerable strain on the principal caregiver and must be resolved at all costs. Sometimes the build-up of losses and stress become too much to bear; often it is the simplest thing that may cause the dam to burst.

Nothing replaces the family relationship.

Careful scheduling is required if the caregiver must mix care provision with work and family responsibilities. Open communication and effective mobilization of all resources can prevent breakdown. Gentle-care recommends seeking professional assistance with legal and financial aspects of guardianship early in the caregiving process. It is

THE UNIQUE GRIEF CYCLE
OF THE CAREGIVER OF PERSONS
WITH DEMENTING ILLNESS

Normal Life

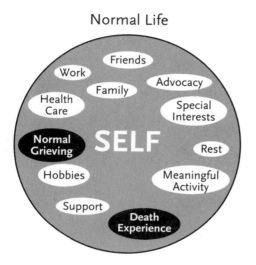

Throughout life we all experience death in one form or another (loss of friend, a job, a pet, etc.). But after an appropriate time of grieving, our life activities return to balance. We continue to give attention to all of the components in our life (family, friends, work, leisure activities, etc.).

FIGURE 16-4

Life While Caregiving for a Person with Dementia

When caregiving someone with dementia, the caregiver *assumes responsibility* for another person. They are surrounded on a daily basis with the "mini" deaths of dementia, and their grief is overwhelming and largely unacknowledged. Other life activities are obliterated by caregiving responsibilities.

FIGURE 16-5

Life After the Death of
Person Under Care

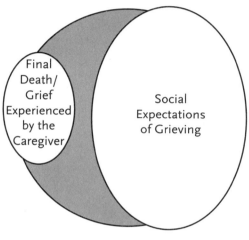

FIGURE 16-6

When physical death finally occurs, the caregiver finds himself alone after years and years of responsibility. They often experience this final death as anticlimactic, or with a sense of relief. Their grief is often muted, since grieving has occurred over many years, and there are few tears left. Society (and other family members), on the other hand, *expect* overt signs of grief, and many misinterpret the feeling of peace, relief, and freedom that the caregiver may exhibit. The caregiver is now faced with the daunting task of beginning to recreate his or her life after a long period of inactivity.

Caregiver's "New" Life

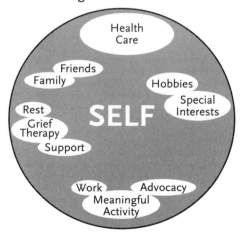

FIGURE 16-7

Persons who wish to help caregivers after the loss of a family member need to help them reconstruct the balance of life activities, with special attention to health issues, grief therapy, and new relationships.

crucially important to remember that no one can provide dementia care alone. Caregivers who learn how to give dementia care and who are supported and loved through the experience remain healthy.

Caregivers' Perceptions of Giving Care

A great deal depends on how the family caregiver perceives the role undertaken. If the caregiver uses maladaptive coping styles, he or she can seriously stress the person with dementia. Overcaring, for example, can cause the sick person to become excessively helpless or very belligerent. Caregivers need to deal with their own feelings surrounding the illness, and may require professional help to do so. Caregiving can be awful, but much of its unpleasantness and stress can be avoided or prevented. Often it's as simple as making a choice: a choice to ask for help; a choice to rest; a choice to simplify a procedure; and a choice to let go of unreasonable expectations.

Caregiver Knowledge Base and Skills

No element of caregiving is as important as that of information and knowledge. Simply put, caregivers who understand dementia give superior care. And they stay healthier.

There are many skills required of the family caregiver. Sometimes skills developed through former experiences are helpful, but often new skills are required to carry out effective dementia care. For example, caregivers must learn how to communicate effectively with someone with temporal lobe brain damage. They must learn how to decipher a "word salad" conversation or complete a dangling sentence. They must learn how to identify and eliminate stress factors affecting the person they are caring for—whether the factor in question is a too-loud TV or a too-complicated place setting. They must learn how to look at problems from all points of view, and find the positive core of each event. For example, in an effort to help, the person with dementia may make a mess or perform poorly. The caregiver must be able to concentrate on the positive motive or intent, rather than the poorly done task.

Reframing is a neuro-linguistic programming technique adopted for Gentlecare. It helps caregivers transform the meaning of behavior. It is a technique for changing the response to certain behaviors to generate new and more satisfying behaviors to choose from. Reframing creates new alternatives. This story illustrates reframing—looking at a situation and finding a different meaning in it:

Adult family homes offer a family ambiance to the person with dementia.

FLORENCE AND ANDY *had been great gardeners. When Andy developed Alzheimer's disease, his wife and family helped him to keep on gardening whenever possible. One day Florence decided to cut down a dead tree on the front lawn and enlisted Andy's help.*

Just as they began the task, Florence was called away to the phone. When she finished her call she found Andy sitting watching TV.

"I thought we were going to get rid of that tree," she said.

"It's done," he replied.

So Florence looked out the window, only to see the dead tree standing straight and tall. On closer inspection she found that their favorite tree, a cherry tree, was all cut up and the wood neatly piled.

Later she said, "Moyra, I had a choice. I could either kill him, or laugh about the whole thing. And I decided it simply wasn't worth getting stressed over."

> On awakening, you look inside your mind and see nothing but black.
>
> —A FAMILY CAREGIVER

One lovely thing that happens when you start telling stories about people with dementia is that it makes you recall all the funny times spent with them. Recalling the story of Andy and Florence and the tree-cutting incident, I'm reminded of another "Andy story."

ONE DAY ANDY AND HIS SON EUGENE were storing stuff in the loft over the carport. Andy was passing the supplies up to Eugene. Suddenly nothing more came up through the hole, so Eugene stuck his head down to see what the delay was. Not only was his father not in sight, but the ladder was gone! Andy had put the ladder neatly away and was watching TV. It was some time before other family members heard faint calls for help and rescued Eugene!

Life Factors Outside of the Illness

The normal responsibilities of life are not suspended when a family member has a dementing illness. Caregivers must add their caregiving responsibilities to what may already be demanding lives.

Spouses and grown children may have full-time work responsibilities—and grown children often have children of their own to look after. People have homes that must be kept up, and many have community commitments that mean a great deal to them. The financial expense of care for a family member may be worrisome, and may add to the burden of care. Family caregivers are often called on to advocate on behalf of the sick person, and this takes courage and diplomacy.

But as we have seen, there can be a way out of burnout and despair. *There can be life after dementia!*

No one can provide dementia care alone!

Those who love or admire family caregivers can assist in the rebuilding of life after the death of a spouse from Alzheimer's, and that assistance is needed both before and after the person's death. A caregiver needs to maintain skills, friendships, and community roles throughout the illness of a family member, and moreover, needs to be without feelings of guilt in doing so. Friends and family are potent agents in helping caregivers achieve these goals, but they need to understand that an exhausted caregiver may not be able to reach out for help. Friendship must be offered, sometimes over and over again.

Caregivers need diversion from their caregiving duties. Special activities such as respite opportunities, vacations, overnight visits, and retreats can refresh and energize a caregiver in amazing ways. It is important to remember, however, that caregivers may require assistance to take advantage of such opportunities.

Few illnesses associated with aging are as devastating to the sick person and his family as dementia. Those who wish to help caregivers can contribute significantly by supporting, reinforcing, and respecting their life relationships and the role of the family. They can help caregivers acquire the support, therapy, and knowledge they need to succeed with this incredible responsibility.

And in partnership with them, we can assist the person with Alzheimer's disease to live as comfortably as possible through the experience.

Professional Care Providers as Therapeutic Agents

In a time of diminishing economic resources for health care services, nothing could be more important than taking a good hard look at the most important resource of all: the people of the health care system. Doing so requires us to think about people in new and different ways to examine their activities with different goals in mind.

It is really amazing what people can do when you let them.

—GORDON FORWARD, CEO, CHAPPARAL STEEL

For most leaders and planners in health care, this requires a paradigm shift—a change in the organizing principle that underlies the way we think about workers in health care, as well as the way services are provided.

Management guru Tom Peters, author of *In Search of Excellence*, says, "There are no limits to the ability to contribute on the part of a properly selected, well trained, appropriately supported and above all, committed person." To paraphrase, average health care workers are capable of moving mountains—if only we ask them to do so and construct a supportive environment for them to work in. Current health care practices raise some vital questions:
- What criteria is used to select workers?
- What is the quality of direction and support being given workers?
- What are the resources workers need to get the job done effectively?

- Where is the opportunity for workers to contribute ideas about how to do the job better?

The paradigm of hierarchy—the pyramid or classic organizational chart—has up to now informed the way most people think and work throughout the health care system. Within that paradigm, authority (i.e., wisdom) flows from the top down to workers at the bottom, who simply carry out directives received from above. This system works exceedingly well in emergencies, but it no longer serves the complex social circumstances in which health care finds itself today.

No system that limits most people while giving power to a few, fosters competition and territoriality, and limits patterns of action to a formula or set pattern can thrive in a world where everything is subject to change and almost everything seems possible. Some of us even believe we can regenerate the old medical paradigm of health care into a new, more effective model. The most obvious motivating force for a new paradigm in health care is the dramatic change being forced on health care systems by our aging population.

Finding a professional caregiver who understands is priceless.

The new model of health care needs to be a cyclical paradigm rather than an hierarchical one. It must embody *interdependence* between the person who is ill and all of us who wish to help, between the afflicted person and his family, and between the care systems and the communities they serve. In her autobiography, *Revolution From Within,* Gloria Steinem speaks of "progress becoming mutual support and connectedness. Progress means interdependence." She proposes an image of an organizational structure that is a circle at rest, and a spiral at work. The cyclical paradigm becomes interdependence.

Old-fashioned hierarchies, in which a few people at the top wield power, a lot of people in the middle wait for orders, and many more at the bottom feel powerless and resentful, are everywhere being challenged as inappropriate and cumbersome. The shift is toward smaller, more lateral and cooperative work units, often known as self-directed work teams. These units are perceived as a breakthrough system for increasing productivity, sparking innovation, and reducing costs.

The fierce competition for power, money, and status, which has always been a major force in health care, is shifting to the practice of trust, respect, and cooperation. The excitement of learning together, appreciating other people's insights, finding effective solutions together, feeling pleasure in cooperative effort, sensing the joy of truly helping people with dementia live more comfortably: the power of these experiences is beginning to chip away at old practices. Each person is beginning to be seen as a unique and capable contributor to effective health care.

The absurd man is he who never changes.

—BARTHÉLÈMY

A circle needs no beginning.

—OLD JAPANESE
PROVERB

AS THE HOUSEKEEPER *for C wing during the first month of Gentlecare, I admit I began a little unsure and apprehensive. In the first two weeks there were a lot of kinks to be improved out, but I must tell you I have come to love it!*

Although it is a busy wing with lots to be done, the new approach has given me a great new sense of fulfillment in my job. I no longer just scrub toilets and mop floors, but have the opportunity to bless the residents such as Sally, simply by letting her help me make the bed or bringing her into the hall to help me dust, when she normally never comes out. To be able to have the opportunity to transform such an anxious person into a happy participating individual, even for a few minutes, is very rewarding for me.

Thank you, Gentlecare, and keep on keeping on.

—*Pat Rankin*
Housekeeper, 1993

Gerontology, or care of the elderly, has always suffered from an image problem: it is perceived by others and sometimes by gerontological practitioners themselves as acute care medicine's poor step-sister. An element of authenticity, of pride in the work done in support of older

CHAPTER
SIXTEEN

people, has always been missing. And gerontological work has always been considered easier than acute care. The qualifications of workers are not assessed as stringently as are those of the workers entrusted with the lives of critical patients. If a person liked old people and had always been kind to grandparents, the person would be considered for employment in gerontology. The practice of gerontology lacked the urgency of more emergency-oriented services. Environment, equipment, and supplies were never truly critical issues, so resources were negotiable. Hanging over all gerontological practice has always been the evil influence of ageism: "Why bother? They are old."

I REMEMBER WORKING ONCE *in the long-term care section of an acute care hospital. From time to time, whenever there was a shortage of physiotherapists in the acute care section, I would be asked to send our gerontology physiotherapist to work in acute care. When I protested that we needed his services, I would be told, "But surely it won't matter if old people miss a few treatments."*

One of the most frequently cited problems in the care of nursing home patients with dementia is the lack of staff knowledge about dementia.

—U.S. CONGRESS, OFFICE OF TECHNOLOGY ASSESSMENT

The new reality of gerontological care flies in the face of such negativism. Anyone who has worked a shift recently in any long-term care facility can attest to the complexity and diversity of the challenges one encounters. With evolving specialization in the management of the diseases of aging has come an awareness that the traditional tools of the medical trade, drugs and surgery, simply do not work in dealing with gerontological problems. The needs of elderly people are changing the practice of medicine. Practitioners are faced with complex social issues that require a body-mind, psycho-social approach to care unlike any previously attempted in Western medical history. There is an urgent need to look beyond symptoms to the context of illness: to considerations of stress, society, family, diet, living arrangements, activity, and emotions.

In that context, the people we choose to work in health care make all the difference. What are their attitudes toward elderly people? What is their level of dedication, their stamina, their professional preparation?

Can we give them the knowledge, skills, and resources to do the job required of them? It behooves us to choose excellent people, and then cherish them and LISTEN TO THEM when they tell us about the world in which they work.

What Qualities Should Staff Members Have?

Since staff members who work with people with dementing illness are therapeutic agents, it is vital that they want to work with this type of client. As we have seen, dementia care depends on the ability of staff members to connect with people afflicted with dementia. Consequently, staff who place a higher priority on accomplishing tasks rather than connecting, or who simply don't want to make the effort to meet people's needs over and over again, should not be assigned to dementia care units—irrespective of seniority, shift priorities, family schedules, health issues, etc. If a staff member does not enjoy dementia care, assigning her to a special care unit will be disastrous for the clients and others working with them. I do not know about others, but I would rather work all alone on a dementia unit than work with someone who does not want to be there.

In providing care for elderly people, it is not just a matter of knowing how something should be done, but rather of knowing how something should be done and doing it that way. Staff members assigned to dementia care units should have, as a minimum, current core training in—

- progressive dementing illnesses
- psychiatric diseases
- physical diseases of aging
- communication, verbal and non-verbal
- problem-solving
- task analysis and age-appropriate programming
- family caregiver relations
- strategies for working with volunteers
- how to develop programs and environments as therapy

Choosing Staff

So how do we choose people who have the qualities needed to deliver excellent dementia care?

The Gentlecare system looks for the following characteristics and background in choosing staff members:

Attitude and beliefs

By this we mean the way a staff member regards someone with dementia, and the way they react to them. It refers to the association of ideas the person has developed through life experience with respect to both old age and dementia. Attitude is the outward manifestation of the principles we hold dear, the convictions and sentiments that inform our actions. As well, people must have enough self-confidence to be effective advocates for those in their care.

Use of language

> *There are no obsolete people, just obsolete skills.*
>
> —FREDRICK HERTZBERG

The way we use language in dementia care is critical, since language shapes the way we act and often the way others act as well. Language must be clear, fair, and objective. It must be used carefully so as not to diminish people. For instance, if someone refers to an old man as violent, that man will be approached in a very different way than if he was said to be upset or frightened.

Preparation

The treatment of progressive dementing illness has only relatively recently become a medical specialty. Staff trained in the biomedical model of care or the psychiatric model of care do not necessarily have the required knowledge base for delivery of good dementia care. In fact, many practitioners speak of the need for such people to unlearn old-style care practices to carry out effective dementia care.

Ongoing- and self-learning is essential to dementia care.

Staff who want to specialize in dementia care require specialized clinical preparation. Since this area of knowledge is still developing, such training must be ongoing. It is important to note that Gentlecare recommends cross-functional training of all staff, volunteers, and family members.

Experience

All of us at one time or another have been children or have helped children develop, so we know what the developmental process is like. Dementia care requires that we learn to understand the reverse of that process and how to support people as they lose skills and functioning. The more positive the life experiences we have had with elders, the more effective we are in supporting them through dementia.

Knowledge

The knowledge base about dementia is changing rapidly. Staff must understand the normal aging processes, the diseases that result in dementia, mental health issues, as well as innovative strategies of care. And learning must be continuous! Gerontological care staff members need to become self-learners.

Skills

Dementia care requires staff members to have skills different from those generally needed in the provision of health care. Strategies or approaches used elsewhere in the health care system are only occasionally appropriate in caring for people experiencing progressive dementia. Specifically, dementia care practitioners require the following skills:

- communication
- problem-solving
- task analysis and presentation
- observation
- stress identification and reduction
- reframing
- distraction
- and more!

One should govern people as one would cook fish, poking as little as possible.

—LAO TZU

Respect

Gentlecare looks for staff members who understand how difficult it is to live with dementia. Respect for brave older people is fundamental to the Gentlecare approach, so staff members must have an intrinsic understanding of the courage and spirit of the people they are helping.

Sense of humor and buoyancy

Despite the huge difficulties it presents, dementia care also offers wonderful opportunities for joy. People with dementia, properly supported, are very funny people who can make you feel very special. It really helps if staff members approach their work with a sense of fun and anticipation rather than a grumpy attitude. Furthermore, a happy demeanor in a staff member changes the way a person with dementia responds.

Designing the Shift

Good dementia care is based on a staff member's ability to enter into therapeutic relationships, to use skills and knowledge to support dysfunctional people, and to develop a prosthetic arrangement of programs and space for each individual in care and the families of those people.

Does this sound like something you can do non-stop for 12 hours? Does this sound like something you can do for a day or two, and then go to a different area in the facility to perform a different job? The job of providing care to persons with dementia is so challenging and complex that the issue of extended shifts and days off must be addressed realistically. It is unrealistic for staff to be able to relate emotionally to a wide variety of people and the public for 12-hour periods. Facilities that schedule staff for this type of shift need to be aware that caregiver burnout is just as prevalent among professional caregivers as it is among family caregivers.

Furthermore, staff members who work 12-hour shifts have long periods of time when they are not on duty. This means that if these staff members are to know what is happening in the lives of the people in care, then they and everyone they work with must have an enormous

Knowledge is not power. Applied knowledge is power.

—ERNIE TADLA,
THE BUSINESS
EXAMINER

One day with a great teacher is better than a thousand days of study.

—OLD CHINESE
SAYING

commitment to information catch-up. It is far too common for staff not to have necessary information about the people they care for, such as changes in functioning levels, strategies, or activities to avoid, information on family dynamics, etc.

AS A DEMENTIA CARE CONSULTANT, *I often approach a staff member who is dressing someone or assisting a person with eating and ask simple questions: How long has this person been here? Does the family visit? How much dinner can this person eat without help?*

It is not unusual for me to receive the response, "You'll have to check at the desk: I just got assigned here from another ward and I've been off duty for several days."

If people acting as therapeutic agents do not know basic information about people in their care, then they certainly can't deliver individualized prosthetic care.

Staff Assignment

The rotation of professional staff in and out of specially designated dementia care areas is another contentious issue. The problems created by 12-hour shift work are identical to those stemming from staff rotation.

Quality dementia care depends first of all on the relationship between staff members, the person with dementia, and the person's

family; secondly, it depends on the knowledge and skill base of staff. Ideally all staff in a long-term care facility would be in a position to deliver prosthetic care, but this is rarely the case. For this reason alone, it is critical to have a stable work group within a dementia care unit.

Gentlecare advocates that a core group of staff sufficient in number to provide care 24 hours a day for a seven-day week be designated as the dementia care team. This group should be permanently assigned to the dementia unit and given responsibility for developing the prosthetic macro-environment.

Once this core group has been established, it becomes possible to

If someone does something extraordinarily well, videotape them at work, and share it with all staff as a study tool.

accept new or rotating staff members into the group, with appropriate orientation and training. Such an arrangement also allows dementia care staff to take time off dementia care assignments for periods of time, for career reasons or when personal issues make it difficult for them to interact in such an intense atmosphere.

Training and Development

Only connect.

—E.M. FORSTER

Knowledge is the key to successful dementia care. The more all staff members know about dementia, the easier and more effective their work becomes. The more family caregivers know, the more willing they are to participate in care, and the more capable they are in supportive roles.

Inservice must be ongoing and involve everyone.

A training program, for example, is used to give staff information about a specific topic, such as how to operate a dishwasher, do a lift, or prepare or serve a meal. Staff development, however, occurs when knowledge is internalized, creating a behavioral change that produces a positive result in both attitude and action. Development is a process, not an event. Development realizes potential; it stimulates growth and change. It releases powers inherent in people so that they strive for effectiveness and excellence.

Training is knowing how to do something. Development is doing it. For example, training is knowing how to put ingredients together into a meal that will meet nutritional needs. Development is presenting that meal to elderly people in a pleasing, serene environment; communicating with them; responding to their concerns; and whenever possible, involving them in food choices and the food preparation process, or in clean-up. Training is knowing how to get eight people up and dressed in time for breakfast, while development is understanding each person's wake-up preferences and performance level; orienting people to time and place; assisting them with their grooming and dressing; and preparing them for and supporting them in the day ahead. These differences in approach are not time related, but rather attitude- and knowledge-based.

Involving Everyone

Health care practice often involves confrontation, competition, and exclusion of various groups of people. Often, information is controlled by a small group in order to enhance the power of that group over others. Territories are developed by one category of staff, and others are not welcome in the space defined by the members of that category. Nursing stations are an example of this.

To provide quality dementia care effectively and efficiently, we have to change the way we think and work so that all types of workers, volunteers, and families can contribute. Involvement is the regular, spontaneous taking of initiative. It is the process of looking at work differently—not in terms of "It's not my job," but rather, "Which of us can do this job best?"

In dementia care, an elderly person may reach out to anyone for help, regardless of that person's academic preparation or job description. This means that the maintenance staff, the hairdresser, and the food service worker must be as well prepared to respond to a request for help as any other team member. In the eyes of the dysfunctional person, the person who is asked for help is the best one. For instance, if the nearest staff member at dinner is addressed with a remark like:

When we see how funny we are, we see how dear we are.

—ANNE WILSON SCHAEFF

- "Where am I?"
- "Have the horses been fed?"
- "I've got to get the hay in!"
- "Someone is killing me!"
- "She stole my glasses!"
- "You can't go in there."

it is simply not appropriate, in dementia care, to say, "Ask the nurse."

In Gentlecare units, in all types of staff members who understand dementing illness and have acquired specialized communication skills, we find superb therapeutic agents. Furthermore, support staff

How can you get very far,
If you don't know who you are?

If you don't know what you've got?
And if you don't know which to do,
of all the things in front of you?

Then what you'll have when you get through
Is just a mess without a clue,
Of all the best that can come true
If you know what and which and who.

— A.A. Milne,
Winnie-the-Pooh

people say that they find that such interaction enhances and enriches their daily work.

That's what learning is. You suddenly understand something you've understood all your life, but in a new way.

—DORIS LESSING

Involvement means sharing information and skills. Some favorite Gentlecare ways of doing this are—

- holding regular open meetings;
- creating communication books that everyone writes in;
- instituting interdisciplinary rounds run on a democratic model;
- proving cross-training and development workshops for all staff;
- role-modeling dementia strategies and approaches;
- using videos;
- using multi-media materials;
- setting up journal clubs; and
- providing exchange locations for articles, write-ups, texts, and journals in communal rooms such as staff rooms or bathrooms.

Involvement means exchanging stifling bureaucratic structures for an environment in which people feel comfortable taking whatever initiative is required to fix problems and extend first-rate service. This does not mean that everyone does everyone else's job! Rather, it implies a healthy respect for and trust in one's colleagues, and an enhanced awareness of each staff person's unique potential.

Building the Team

Health care institutions have traditionally held interdisciplinary rounds in which the members of divergent professions meet to discuss the status and plans for those in their care. Following such meetings, each professional representative then goes to practice in isolation from the other members of the team. This sort of exercise has resulted in a focus on power allocation and territoriality rather than care.

Example is leadership.

—ALBERT SCHWEITZER

For example, it is not unusual for staff to compete for client time: rehabilitation, recreation, and activities staff schedule their care strategies at times when care staff do not "need" the sick person whether or not those times are appropriate for the person in care. Similarly, food service personnel often decide on the timing of residents' meals, even if the times selected are incompatible with their comfort or with care plans that nurses have developed. Only rarely are support personnel, housekeeping, maintenance, and food service staff included in team rounds, and even then it is usually as observers rather than as full working participants.

Teamwork, on the other hand, involves much more synergy. Teams are democratic, autonomous, highly trained, and have responsibility for problem-solving and for formulating effective care delivery systems. They must work together, not just talk together. The team leader is often the best facilitator, not the most highly trained person.

Good leaders make all the difference.

The Leader's Job

In the new paradigm of care, the role of the team leader (coordinator, unit manager) is completely transformed. It encompasses helping the group articulate a vision and a set of values; group facilitation; people development; quality control; planning; coordination; and creation of a flexible, responsive support system. The leader's focus moves from one of being directive to one of ensuring participation. Tom Peters describes this as a change from "cop to facilitator" or "management by walking around." Of course, such a shift requires that such leaders or coordinators acquire the skills needed to do the job differently.

The use of 12-hour shifts, seconded from acute medical practice, does not work in dementia care.

Changing Organizational Style and Structure

Gentlecare advocates a review of traditional organizational structures that emphasize extreme specialization and job definition. The power of well-chosen, well-trained, well-supported people working in team-based management is so awesome it is breathtaking. Top-down management style is simply too unresponsive and cumbersome to be practical in gerontological care.

It is easy to put people down. It is harder to lift them up.

In traditionally structured long-term care facilities, the people who have been entrusted with decision-making are frequently simply not available when action needs to be taken. (This is not true in most acute care treatment situations where the physician as team leader is usually on hand to make critical decisions.) In long-term care, whoever makes the critical contact with the cognitively impaired client or his family must be in a position to respond positively.

THIS REMINDS ME OF A TIME *when an extended care unit reported a problem with swallowing disorders. When I reviewed the unit's feeding procedure, I noticed that staff members used large soup spoons to feed people. I suggested that a small spoon might be less intrusive, and might reduce the possibility of gagging and choking. The staff agreed and said they had asked for small spoons, but the big spoons kept coming up on the trays. I asked whom they had contacted, and they said they had asked their supervisor to check with the dietician, to see if she would ask her supervisor to discuss the matter with the director of care, who presumably could raise the matter with her administrative counterpart. Eight months later, big spoons were still causing swallowing problems.*

Gentlecare addresses the challenge of developing quality care by shifting from a hierarchical management style to decentralized, team-based management. The following criteria are built into the management program:

- staff specialization within interdisciplinary, self-managing teams
- adjustments in jurisdictions
- participation by all
- skill enhancement for everyone
- rewarding of initiative
- empowerment of workers, families, and volunteers

Building a Community:
Volunteers as Care Providers

Volunteers are not staff! Volunteers do not do staff work. Volunteers are not replacements for professional staff. Rather, volunteers have a critical and unique role to play in health care delivery that cannot be undertaken by paid workers.

Volunteers are tangible links to the outside, and are not part of the health service community. They are normal, ordinary people, and representative of the dozens of people we all interact with in our daily lives. They evoke memories of times past, good times, and healthy periods in life. They are the bridge between health care institutions and ordinary life. For people suffering from dementia, for whom life in the community has been abruptly truncated, volunteers provide a comforting link to a time that was important, joyful, and under their own control. No matter how diligently staff try, they cannot achieve this sense of naturalness in their relationships with residents, since their work inevitably casts them in a different role, with a different set of functions. Gentlecare regards volunteers as therapeutic partners in creating systems that are comforting and prosthetic for vulnerable elderly people. In such a

It is one of the most beautiful compensations in life that no man can sincerely try to help another without helping himself.

—EMERSON

One in four Canadians perform volunteer work.

partnership, there is no limit to what can be achieved. Without volunteers there is no possibility that staff alone can create an environment that meets the needs of dementia sufferers.

Throughout the world, volunteers contribute to organizations in myriad ways: fund-raising, direct service, research, transportation, one-on-one visiting, entertainment, education, advocacy, contribution of specialized skills, liaison, emergency assistance, ombudsman service, service to voluntary boards, support groups, activators, organizers, and catalysts... the list is endless.

Do these activities sound like tasks that need to be done to support dementia care? Do these activities sound like tasks that professional staff are in a position to undertake? If any one of these activities were undertaken in a dementia care unit, would the workload be eased? Would dysfunctional elderly people be comforted? I think so. I know so. Gentlecare units that work in partnership with volunteers cannot imagine operating without them.

I do it for myself.

—A VOLUNTEER

In Canada, 5.3 million people contribute their time in formal organizations, and 13 million people help in informal ways. Volunteers have many redeeming characteristics, but in these days of shrinking economic resources they have one enchanting quality: volunteers are an infinite resource!

Volunteers are available in unlimited numbers. There is no "cap," no predetermined "F.T.E.," no budget restriction, no resource allocation. Organizations can have as many volunteer partners as they can accommodate comfortably and effectively. There is no task that someone, somewhere, somehow in the community cannot accomplish. The secret lies in simply asking.

I REMEMBER WORKING *with a group of elderly veterans. When any one of these old gentlemen left the hospital, his belongings would be packed either in a garbage bag or a cardboard box. Somehow this just seemed a bit tacky. A phone call to the local Royal Canadian Legion Ladies Auxiliary explaining the problem elicited this response: "Give us a little while." Within hours, a car drove up and discharged a mass of suitcases in different sizes and shapes "for the boys." I can still re-member the delight this generous gift brought, and the difference it made at discharge time.*

Volunteers are vital links that keep whole communities together. Volunteers are communities! And they can help us build the vital alternate or surrogate mini-community required to help people with dementing illness live through the disease. Without volunteers—

- Who speaks for your community?
- Who supports families in crisis?
- Who helps create a sense of home and familiarity for our sick elders?
- Who gathers community resources to address urgent needs?
- Who provides the beauty, the music, the spiritual comfort?
- Who goes for walks and takes time to talk?
- Who offers comfort in the dying time?
- Who reads?
- Who has the time?
- Who makes the cups of tea?
- Who knows how things used to be?
- Where are the young with their laughter and their enthusiasm?
- Who do you call when you have a crisis?

In Gentlecare programs, it's volunteers—that's who!

Planning for Volunteering

But good volunteer programs don't just happen. Volunteers do not come out of the walls by osmosis. Volunteer involvement in health care requires careful planning and nourishing. Volunteers are motivated by many factors:

- the wish to learn;
- the hope to do something successfully;
- the new experience;
- the desire to give of oneself;

- the need to exert power and influence;
- the desire to problem-solve;
- the wish to advocate for favorite causes;
- the desire to have fun, to make a difference;
- the urge to meet new people and friends;
- the opportunity to be creative;
- the wish to acquire skills and knowledge; and
- the desire to be useful and competent.

And almost everyone wants to do a good job.

Volunteer systems can be divided into four areas of focus:

Recruitment

The acquisition of volunteers is everyone's business. Although they may be formally welcomed into the organization by a coordinator of volunteers, everyone needs to be on the lookout for suitable candidates. Once volunteers are attracted to the unit, Gentlecare recommends that they be invited to a one-to-one placement interview. During the interview, the volunteer's motivation, skills, and needs can be identified. A volunteer assignment sheet can be completed, and a preliminary placement discussed. Gentlecare advocates an initial trial placement, with an option for either party to renegotiate. The volunteer should leave the interview with a clear understanding of the assignment, the commitment of both parties, and the organizational system within which he will be working.

Would-be volunteers who do not meet organizational criteria should be referred elsewhere. Do not send them to a care unit to see how it works out. This can sabotage the whole volunteer program. If there are any reservations about the suitability of a volunteer, ask the person to work under supportive supervision for a trial period.

Volunteers can be recruited from social or service organizations, seniors centers, universities, colleges, high schools, church groups, special interest groups, talent pools, ethnic groups—anywhere, actually, where people are to be found.

Education

Like any person on staff, volunteers must know what they are doing, and which actions are or are not appropriate. Gentlecare recommends cross-training of volunteers with staff, that is, the inclusion of volunteers in any staff education or development activities. This can be a valuable experience for both groups, and can develop important bonding for work with those in care. In addition to that training, volunteers need to understand how the organization works; who does what; who they can count on for help; confidentiality; and appropriate responses.

They also must learn effective communication skills prior to assignment. Do not send new volunteers to a unit to talk to patients. This is terrifying! The volunteers will disappear and never come back! Instead, suggest they work in partnership with an experienced volunteer until they feel comfortable on their own.

Ongoing education

This is a sure-fire way to engage and retain volunteers. If the process of dementing illness is explained to them, if they understand the behavior it causes, and if they are taught effective strategies and approaches, they will be hooked forever. The strategies used in dementia care make sense to volunteers: they are do-able and they make elderly people who are ill feel wonderful. All these elements make for a successful volunteer experience.

If we want to help people change, it's important that we don't push them or pull them— just walk together.

Support

The job of volunteer coordinator is to make sure everyone knows what each volunteer is doing within the organization. *But supporting volunteer efforts is everyone's job.* It is critical that everyone greets volunteers, acknowledges their assignments, helps direct and support them, and thanks them. In order to contribute effectively, volunteers need to feel welcome. It is so very sad, and such a waste, to see volunteers tiptoeing around professional territories, afraid to make a mistake. Would any of us volunteer under such circumstances? Would we feel confident and successful? Support can come in many forms, but as a minimum, each contact person within the organization should say to each volunteer:

- "It's great to have you here."
- "We notice a difference when you visit."
- "Your help is really appreciated."
- "Thanks for coming."

Regular, honest, helpful feedback is also a source of encouragement to volunteers, as it is to everyone! Don't tell volunteers what not to do; tell them what you need to have them do to help you or the client, and if necessary show them how to do it.

Acknowledgement

Volunteers don't expect to be paid, but like any human being, they appreciate having their contributions acknowledged. I have worked in organizations that have celebrated volunteers with a huge gala dinner or party. These events are costly, take endless hours of staff time to organize, and usually end with everyone wondering if it was worth all the fuss and bother. Gentlecare rather recommends ongoing acknowledgement of volunteers in any of the following ways:

- providing an introduction in the organization's newsletter, or posting notices on the bulletin board;
- publicizing the "volunteer idea of the month" or "contribution of the month";
- sending notes of appreciation for special accomplishments;
- making brief presentations to the board of directors or the executive committee reporting on outstanding work; and
- ensuring acceptance of the volunteer as a valuable member of the team.

Gentlecare believes that volunteers are so vital to dementia care that the position of Coordinator of Volunteers should be a full-time responsibility, rather than an add-on to some other job.

A Word About Groups of Volunteers

For social and support reasons, volunteers from large service organizations often prefer to visit institutions in groups. This practice is very intimidating for elderly people, and overwhelming for staff on duty. Often staff attention has to be focused on caring for the volunteers rather than on the people in their care. As well, volunteer groups sometimes expect unrealistic levels of participation on the part of residents and staff.

> I REMEMBER WORKING *on a dementia unit one evening, and becoming aware that the ward staff had rounded up some very impaired elderly people and grouped them around the elevator. When I inquired about what was happening, I was told that it was Rotary bingo night, and that the bingo volunteers always expected a large turnout. Very sick elderly people who couldn't even recognize a bingo card if you paid them were being used to meet perceived expectations.*
>
> *This is wrong, but it is also a very common occurrence. Staff are placed in the untenable position of knowing such activity is harmful to their clients, but feeling powerless to object for fear of offending very important volunteers.*

It is the care facility's responsibility to clearly outline the needs of its clients, and to specify what help is appropriate. No service organization worth its salt should insist on doing something harmful to people. In most cases, they are only doing what they think is best, or re-creating something that they have done for years for another client group (and which no one has talked to them about re-defining).

Gentlecare recommends that large service organizations be invited to have their volunteers visit in pairs (two people, that is!), or if they prefer, they may work together as a group *outside the facility* to accomplish a specific task such as letter writing, shawl making, Christmas present wrapping, and fund-raising.

A Further Word about Volunteer Auxiliaries

Over the years, hospital auxiliaries have made magnificent contributions to health care. They are often a source of donations of both money and specific equipment. Traditionally, they have also operated services such as tuck shops, gift shops, and beauty parlors. Auxiliaries are usually associated with acute care hospitals rather than long-term care facilities.

With the tremendous increase in the numbers of people with dementia that are appearing in health care institutions, it becomes advisable for the members of auxiliaries to participate in educational programs developed for individual volunteers. For example, auxiliaries frequently get involved in decorating health care facilities; in dementia care units, this work can be greatly enhanced if the importance of environmental adaptation is explained to the participants.

Family Members as Volunteers

Family members often ask to volunteer their services or simply assume volunteer jobs in the course of caring for their family members. Often this is enormously helpful to people with dementia, staff, and the family caregiver. After all, relatives know the problems very well, and have definite ideas about the quality of care that should be offered.

However, it is important to note that in an effort to expiate their guilt and grief, some family members or caregivers nearly live in the facility day and night. These people are already exhausted and in no position to approach people with dementia in a therapeutic way. Staff members need to work with these caregivers to help them focus attention on their own needs and grief.

Volunteers are an infinite resource!

Family members who volunteer should be registered, trained, and supported just like any other volunteer; being a dementia caregiver doesn't automatically qualify someone for a volunteer assignment. Often their interest can be directed to advocacy or fund-raising, to give them some relief from the grind of personal care. Sometimes it is helpful to match family caregivers with volunteers who have the time and energy to listen and be there for them, and to help them in advocating appropriately for their family member in care. Family volunteers must be assessed carefully on an ongoing basis for exhaustion and burnout.

SOMETIMES VOLUNTEERS HELP OUT *in unexpected ways. In one facility everyone was concerned about the ugly, uncomfortable dining room on the dementia care unit. Staff members were at their wits' end wondering how they could improve the ambiance. They responded to the suggestion to ask the volunteer auxiliary to develop a suitable environment. Working together they created a simply lovely, comfortable room where elderly people felt at home. The last time we spoke, they were beginning to work on the bathrooms.*

Do not send new volunteers to a unit "to talk to patients."

And Others...

Sometimes staff members themselves volunteer in lovely ways. At one facility in Ontario, Larry, one of the housekeeping staff members, brings in his new baby to visit one evening each week. The event is called "Larry's Baby Night," and is a highlight of the activity schedule.

In developing dementia care services, it is critical that we establish a vital link with volunteers and community organizations. We need to look closely at the unique and priceless contribution that only volunteers can bring to health care. We need to recognize the contribution of volunteers as social change agents, as problem solvers, and as prudent managers of resources.

We need to stop regarding volunteers as charming extras, as peripheral assets—nice, but non-essential. Perhaps we need to stop recognizing them one week in every year, and begin to realize that we need them every day of the year if we hope to meet the needs of today's sick people.

17

Working Together in Therapeutic Partnership

She's not my caregiver,
she's my wife!
　　　　　—man with Alzheimer's disease

The experience of working with people suffering from Alzheimer's disease or a related dementia is challenging, and often filled with despair. But there are moments of insight and clarity that open new pathways for direction or action. More often than not, this new way of thinking is inspired by the people experiencing the disease, rather than by those who only observe their struggle.

The quote at the head of this chapter—the plaintive cry of a husband: "She's not my caregiver, she's my wife!"—occurred during one of the moments that opened up my thinking. I was listening as a professional staff member explained to the man that his wife had been his caregiver, but now she was tired. Now, they—the facility staff members—would be his new caregivers. His wife was going home to rest. His point, of course, was that this was not a question of merely substituting caregivers, as one might substitute a team player in the middle of a game—but rather that we were separating him from his *wife*. Implicit in his cry was the conviction that no one of us could ever replace her. She was his WIFE!

Family members have always held a place of importance in the health care systems I have designed: they are a source of vital information, they help their loved ones feel good, and they often help out during various programs. But this man was talking about something far more significant. He was saying that in addition to being his caregiver, his wife was his life partner, his soul mate, maybe his best friend, and definitely his major support system. In that moment, it became clear to me that the prescribed role we have developed for the significant family member in health care is not appropriate within dementia care.

The expected role of the spouse or family member is to visit two or three times each week, chat briefly with their loved one, provide some special food treat, and share concerns while we share our observations with her. This places the spouse in the role of "hospital visitor" rather than partner and diminishes their importance. This ritual, played out day after weary day, does not serve the person with dementia well, nor does it offer support to family members. This approach not only fails to alleviate the guilt and grief of the family, it frequently exacerbates those feelings.

For staff members, family visits simply add one more task to an already busy day. If the family is pleased with the service that is being provided, the visit can be a pleasant interlude. If the family is upset or, perish the thought, in advocacy mode, the burden for staff becomes intolerable.

Certain health care systems simply do not allocate appropriate time for staff to meet with families and develop effective working relationships. Staff members often do not understand issues of caregiving or the grief and pain associated with institutionalizing a family member. Complaints about institutional inadequacies are often taken as personal criticisms. Professional staff sometimes do not acknowledge the legal responsibilities of families nor their role as advocates. Families are often referred to as "the second client," while no provision is made in staff schedules to work with families.

Gentlecare views the significant family member (often the spouse) as the *principal caregiver,* whether the person with dementia lives at home or in a facility. The person who is established in the mind of the person experiencing dementia as the central support person is the principal caregiver. All others who seek to help must do so in sec-

Every day he is slowly dying, and part of me is dying with him.

—A SPOUSE

ondary roles, working always to support and encourage the family member in her arduous role.

If no family member exists, or none is able to assume the role of supporting the sick person, if it is at all possible someone must be found within the staff or volunteer community to serve as a surrogate family member. The person with dementia must feel that there is someone who is there for him, who can be counted on, who will accept him just the way he is, without expectations or judgement.

Professional caregivers often say that their families are absent, exhausted, dysfunctional, or impossible. And this can be true—some families are those things. But by far, the majority of families care deeply about their loved ones. When they fail to express those positive feelings, almost without exception it is because they are experiencing symptoms of caregiver syndrome: extreme fatigue, stress, grief, depression, guilt, poor health, isolation, and burnout. Research has shown that family caregivers reach an emergency state of exhaustion after only two years of caregiving, but most families give care for double or triple that time before seeking help.

It is rare for families to abandon a spouse or parent. With education and support, family members can and do work to achieve a state of comfort and happiness for people experiencing dementia. Because of their history and perspective, they can accomplish things that professional caregivers can never achieve.

Gentlecare seeks to harness this therapeutic potential by developing partnerships with family members both in the home and in facilities. A partnership begins with a written, voluntary contract that clearly outlines the role each party will attempt to play in the life of the person with dementia. It identifies the professional worker who will be the central contact for the person with dementia, and the spokesperson from the family. It outlines concrete ways in which each party will work to support and assist the other to achieve more effective treatment outcomes. In addition to achieving those outcomes, the partnership helps to prevent family caregivers from succumbing to caregiver burnout and illness.

I was out of energy, out of patience, and I was afraid I was out of love, because I was starting to scream at him.

—WIFE-CAREGIVER

The Gentlecare Therapeutic Partnership Contract

Gentlecare designs a contract with families that clearly lays out responsibility.

Family Responsibilities

BE INFORMED

As painful as it may be, family members need information about the disease process their loved one is experiencing. In Gentlecare, families are provided the same educational programs that are delivered to professional staff.

PROVIDE HISTORY

Vital background information about the person with dementia helps staff create the appropriate prosthesis. Such information refers to personality, culture, education, profession, community affiliations, family constellation, habits, skills, interests, idiosyncrasies, spirituality, preferences, and strengths.

IDENTIFY A FAMILY CONTACT PERSON

To ensure effective communication, professional caregivers need to have a family spokesperson identified. As a rule, this person is the spouse or legal guardian.

SPECIFY SERVICES ANTICIPATED

Prior to admission, family caregivers need to discuss their expectations of care with professional staff and physician(s). Issues to be covered in that discussion include at least the following: use of medication, restraints, clothing, nutrition, room partners, activity programs, walking opportunities indoors and outdoors, end of life issues, and so on.

BE HONEST AND OPEN IN COMMUNICATION

Action happens when families talk to the person in the organization who can create change. Complaining to everyone or to no one does not advance the cause of more effective care. Families often feel frightened or impatient when confronted by a faceless organization. They may fear reprisals to their family member if they complain. They are terrified that the person with dementia might be asked to leave the facility if the family raises care issues. However unfounded such fears may be,

Alzheimer's is a terrible, terrible way to die . . . and taking care of people with Alzheimer's is a terrible way to live.

—DR. ALLEN ROSES,
DUKE UNIVERSITY

it is a perception that can immobilize family caregivers. On the other hand, family caregivers sometimes complain about every small detail of care as a way of managing their feelings of guilt for having placed their loved one in an institution. Constant complaints often result in no one paying attention when real concerns surface.

Gentlecare encourages families to make detailed notes of their concerns, making sure to include date, time, and a contact person. Often this process alone helps to clarify issues. Once a concern has been validated, it can be taken to the person responsible for that particular aspect of care for resolution.

Every effort should be made to minimize complaints based on hearsay, non-specific complaints, or uncorroborated claims. Techniques such as avoidance of discussion, stonewalling, power trips, manipulation, scapegoating, and buck-passing should also be discouraged.

A good rule of thumb in the management of complaints is to remember always that families and care providers share the same objective: a decent quality of life for the person in care.

NEGOTIATE THE FAMILY ROLE

Family members need to be candid about their relationships with the person with dementia and the scope of their responsibilities. Spouses may take full charge of care or they may share aspects of responsibility with mid-life children or siblings. Long-distance caregivers may be able to provide financial support but may not be able to visit very often. Family disputes or areas of conflict should be identified. Each family is different, and these differences must be respected in planning for care.

MAKE A TENTATIVE SCHEDULE OF FAMILY VISITS

It is very helpful for facility or home support personnel to know when the family caregiver or some other member of the family is going to be visiting the person with dementia. This information is important.

The common view is that this is because staff want to "fix up" the person prior to the visit. Possibly, but this information is important in Gentlecare because staff members create a different prosthesis if family are present than the one they put in place when the person is alone. Schedules allow both parties to maximize resources and build the day around these important contacts.

Families are advised to spend time with the person in care as often as it is comfortable and healthy for them to do so. Visiting schedules vary from every day, three times per week, weekend visits, brief evening visits, to two to three times per year.

It is very hard to visit someone in hospital. Family caregivers need help in determining how often they can tolerate the stress, both physically and psychologically. If families are confident that good care is in place, they feel more comfortable spacing out their visits.

It is important to work with families to determine the best time of day for them to visit; visiting may be best at the time of awakening, or perhaps at bedtime, or again, may best take the form of a shared walk before dinner. It is often helpful to avoid the times when personal care is being offered, since the person with dementia cannot concentrate on several things at once.

Family contact may be the best therapy we can offer. The schedule of family visits should form the basis of any care plan.

ACCEPT CERTAIN DUTIES ON BEHALF OF A FAMILY MEMBER

Caring for someone with dementia is the most exacting task ever undertaken. When we pool efforts and skills, the burden is lightened for everyone, and better care occurs. Family caregivers should be encouraged and allowed to continue to care for their loved one. Care may take the form of regular walks, massage, hair management, nail care, hydration, clothes management, care of personal effects in rooms, assistance with creating a sense of home in the institution, fund-raising, and advocacy. Some families with help find that they can reach out to other sick people who live with their family member.

BE TOLERANT

Caring for large numbers of people with dementia is a daunting task. Most professional caregivers do the very best they can, but health care systems are complex organizations, and problems inevitably occur. Family members who try to understand the issues, and who work with staff to solve problems, will appreciate the much higher quality of care that results.

ASSIST AND FACILITATE IN THE SEARCH FOR RESOLUTIONS

Once families understand their role and are comfortable with it, there

Come not when I am dead, to drop thy foolish tears upon my grave.

—LORD TENNYSON

is no end to the magic that ensues. In my experience, solutions to most serious problematic behaviors have almost always come as a result of family information and collaboration.

Consider this scenario. The spouse of a man whose nutrition is seriously compromised by dementia comments to staff: "My husband always loved raspberries and ice cream." If staff responds, "Wouldn't we all! But this is not a restaurant," the exchange leaves the family member frustrated, angry, and helpless. If only her husband were at home, she could give him all the things he loves, but he can't be at home because he is too ill. The staff member, exasperated by the seemingly extravagant demands of the family, thinks: "Has she any idea what a facility food budget looks like? It's not my fault he is not eating raspberries. I do the best I can for everyone here."

Let's suppose the staff member had responded differently: "Oh! Do you think he might eat that? We don't have ice cream or berries available, but if you bring them in, I'll mix them in a smoothie for your husband, and we will see if he can manage it. Wouldn't it be wonderful if we could get a good protein drink into him?" This response acknowledges the family member's concern; states the fact that the institution doesn't have special foods readily available; gives the family member a critical role; and joins staff and family together in shared responsibility for helping the person with dementia.

Facility Responsibilities

INFORM
Family caregivers need to understand the disease issues fully as much as do general care staff. Gentlecare units include family members in regular staff in-service and educational sessions. It is also useful to create a special education bulletin board for the public, on which current "Info Bites" are posted. Avoid newspaper clippings with the latest and often unfounded miracle cures, and items that are outdated. Regular family information and support meetings are very helpful as well.

RECEIVE INFORMATION
Families are the major source of vital information about individuals with dementia. Efforts to include families as part of the treatment team

are rewarded over and over again by help in constructing better prostheses.

COMMUNICATE EFFECTIVELY

Families need information and stories about their family member to assuage their pain and guilt, ease their loneliness, and to survive. They do not need to hear horror stories, complaints, or disasters. After all, if they had been able to manage problematic behaviors, the person with dementia never would have been institutionalized in the first place. Furthermore, in today's climate of economic restraint, stories of cutbacks, staff shortages, reduced services, and closures are terrifying for the family caregiver, who dreads harmful changes for the person in care.

IDENTIFY A CONTACT PERSON IN THE FACILITY

The Gentlecare system suggests that each family needs a facility liaison person who is responsible for keeping family members informed, transferring information and stories, listening to complaints, and referring caregivers to appropriate sources of help. This liaison person is responsible for identifying a substitute contact person for the family when the assigned liaison person is not available.

IDENTIFY ROLES/DUTIES FOR THE FAMILY

Families are often frightened or awed by hospital or health care organizations. To make sure that family members are comfortable working in dementia care areas, it is critical that staff members identify items of work in which the help of families would be appreciated.

I remember a situation where a wife asked me, a visiting consultant, "Is it all right if I give my husband a drink of water?"

One facility I know solves the problem by simply posting signs such as: "We need help with the garden. We need books for the living room. Does anyone know where we can get a turkey?"

RESPECT FAMILY CONCERNS AND RESPONSIBILITIES

All staff need to be aware of the family's relationship to the person in care. In Gentlecare we find it useful to review this information at team conferences or when major changes in care plans are contemplated.

UNDERSTAND THE FAMILY'S SORROW

Dementia devastates families! The anxiety, pain, and grief caused by

Oh Moyra! I wish it would end.

—AN ELDERLY CAREGIVER

the progress of the disease are overwhelming; it is not uncommon for family caregivers to feel rage, frustration, and impotence; and whether the person with dementia is institutionalized or at home, the responsibility of the family remains exhausting.

All these factors have an impact on the family members' relationships and interactions. Compassion and empathy from those of us on the sidelines is very helpful.

CONTRACT FOR SPECIFIC SERVICES

Staff members need to be candid and specific in identifying special requirements such as help with bathing, assistance with walking at specific times, and special nutritional needs.

Unresolved complaints help no one ... not the person with the disease, not the family member, nor the staff. Resolutions, on the other hand, are a source of joy for everyone.

Unfortunately, specific requests are unusual; it is more common for a family to hear, "We need someone with the person all the time." The usual result of that kind of request for help is that a person untrained in dementia care is hired by the family to watch the person with dementia. This is an expensive, demoralizing, and ineffectual way to provide dementia care.

IDENTIFY THE INSTITUTION'S ROUTINE AND EXPECTATIONS

It is important to sit down with families and explain the routines, policies, and procedures of the institution. In Gentlecare we do this on an individual basis and in writing, although the information may also be provided during support group meetings or on bulletin boards.

Every family caregiver hears information differently!

ACCEPT THE FAMILY'S COMMITMENT TO THE PERSON IN CARE

For the most part, families are deeply committed to organizing the best quality of life possible for their loved one. It behooves staff members to understand this, and work with the family to achieve this mutual goal.

Joint Responsibilities

RESPECT THE PERSON WITH DEMENTIA AS AN ADULT HUMAN BEING WHO IS DYSFUNCTIONAL

Health care organizations that undertake the care of elderly people with dementia should be held accountable for regarding their clients with respect, as they would any other sick individuals.

DISCOVER THE LEVEL OF ABILITY OF EVERY PERSON WITH DEMENTIA

Appropriate assessment procedures should be undertaken to determine each individual's needs and strengths. Only then can an effective prosthesis be designed.

PROVIDE A PROSTHETIC ENVIRONMENT (PHYSICAL/EMOTIONAL/SPIRITUAL)

Health care organizations that offer care to people with dementia have a responsibility to provide an environment that compensates for physical dysfunction and offers emotional and spiritual care. Families have a responsibility to collaborate in this effort.

APPRECIATE EACH OTHER'S RESPONSIBILITIES

Both family caregivers and professional caregivers have responsibility for the person with dementia. Great care happens when everyone respects the contributions of one another.

SUPPORT AND ASSIST EACH OTHER

Staff often argue that there isn't time to look out for families. In my experience, when help has been extended to families everyone's job is made easier; clients function at higher levels; support for dementia care increases; and staff feel excited about going to work on Monday.

ACKNOWLEDGE THE CONTRIBUTION OF EACH

The exciting health care organizations that I visit acknowledge good work—no matter who does it. They do so through employee-of-the-month citations; caregiver-of-the-month privileged parking; idea-of-the-week recognitions; Gentlecare strategy-of-the-week awards; and volunteer-we-can't-manage-without awards.

COMMUNICATE CANDIDLY AND CARINGLY

Honest, sensitive communication encourages people to perform in outstanding ways and risk failures. Staff should feel comfortable asking families, "How do you think we're doing?" And families should not fear to ask, "What could I do to be more supportive of my family member?"

When stars work in your organization, everyone shines!

TIPS FOR DEVELOPING
A RAPPORT WITH FAMILIES

1. Prior to admission, provide families with an understanding of the facility's philosophy, and always remember the grieving that occurs at the time of placement.

2. Keep admission day simple and low-key. Enjoy a cup of tea with the new resident and family members.

3. Always phone the family the morning after admission to tell them how the first night went.

4. Keep them informed! Encourage phone calls. Initiate phone calls to an ailing caregiver.

5. Set up a buddy system with another appropriate family member.

6. Encourage flexible visiting times and help them understand what is too little or too much for their loved one, depending on the adjustment of the resident.

7. Make a point of talking to every family member when they visit.

8. Provide an area for families to visit comfortably.

9. Help families feel comfortable on the unit and help them adapt to the behavior of other residents.

10. Friendly reminders of the atmosphere we wish to create is sometimes necessary if families visit with active toddlers or large numbers of people.

11. Always make time for a family member.

12. Remember that a complaining family is a hurting family.

13. Encourage participation in a family group.

14. Provide freedom of information.

15. Involve family members in care planning.

16. Provide reassurance regarding appropriate clothing to bring, lost articles, etc.

17. Encourage participation in educational sessions.

18. Help family understand that this is their unit, and encourage participation in projects.

19. Share with families your special moments experienced with their loved one.

20. Send photos to out-of-town family members.

21. Encourage family members to stay for a meal or a special occasion.

FIGURE 17-1

—SANDY TELFORD, RN, DELTAVIEW HABILITATION CENTRE

18

Cherishing the Memory, Living the Reality

To live in the hearts we leave behind is not to die.

For family members the final physical devastation of Alzheimer's disease happens at a time when their resources are virtually depleted. It is hard not to get caught up in the last slow, painful chapter of dementia. Families must watch as one body system after another closes down, and death appears imminent with each labored breath. But as all of us who have sat these vigils know, the human spirit clings tenaciously to life. Sometimes it can seem a lifetime between breaths before the last one.

Families struggle, too, with end-of-life issues: medical intervention or no medical intervention; antibiotics; intravenous feeding and hydration; resuscitation; relief from pain. Each family, with the aid of their advisors, must make these difficult decisions.

During the first six stages of Alzheimer's disease, Gentlecare is focused on correctly identifying and maximizing the afflicted person's remaining strengths. However, in the final stage of the disease, when the mind as we know it is lost, Gentlecare strategies are designed to ensure the comfort of the dying person through hydration, nutrition, massage, spiritual care, and respect. The critical efforts of the Gentlecare program shift: the goal now is to assist and support the family in achieving a serene passage from life to death for their beloved family member.

The family is encouraged and supported in the effort to be with the dying person through the final mysterious stage of life. Family members are helped to reach the person on a sensory level through the use of strategies that include massage, holding, wrapping, rocking, and cradling. Strategies to reach the person on a spiritual level include the use of music, prayer, readings, hymns, and words of endearment. Each activity must be chosen carefully to appropriately reflect the culture of the individual.

Often when there is little or no response from the dying person, family members feel discouraged, grief stricken, or even foolish in their efforts. Those of us in roles of support, whether home support personnel, neighbors, hospice workers, facility staff, or family members, need to role model and encourage efforts to reach the sick person: there is evidence that at some level, the person with dementia can be reached and afforded a sense of peace; and without doubt, families who engage in such activity through the dying time of dementia feel comforted and effective.

Today is a good day to die for all the things in my life are here.

—CHIEF CRAZY HORSE

I WAS PRIVILEGED *to be present at the dying time of a man with whom I had worked as he and his family lived through the experience of dementia. He and I had shared a love of dogs, and had spent many lovely times together swapping stories and playing with my dogs. As he lay curled up in the final stages of life, the grief and loss of his family was devastating. They felt unable to reach him in any way. No vestige of the man they loved remained. With the family's consent, I decided to bring my big basset, Michael, to visit. As the man lay curled up on the bed, we placed the dog in his arms beside him. Big Mike of course loves to cuddle, and made the most of this comfortable place. Gradually as the dog's warmth and softness permeated his skin, the man began slowly, ever so slowly, to stroke the dog's fur. How could this be, when no purposeful movement is possible at this stage? And yet, as the family watched the tiny familiar gesture, they were flooded with memories of their loved one—in different times, in better times. Suddenly he was with us again.*

*Let me not to the marriage of true minds admit
impediments. Love is not love
which alters when it alteration finds,
Or bends with the remover to remove:
Oh No! it is an ever-fixed mark,
that looks on tempests and is never
shaken.*

*It is the star to every wandering bark
whose worth's unknown, although his
height be taken.*

*Love is not Time's fool, though rosy
lips and cheeks within his
bending sickles compass comes;
Love alters not with his brief
hours and weeks
But bears it out even to the edge
of doom.*

*If this be error, and upon
me proved*

*I never write, nor no man
ever loved.*

—William Shakespeare

By far the greatest effort to be made is celebrating the memory of
the person—the person who was, before dementia began its dreadful
course. Families need to be helped to remember, through stories and
pictures, the deeds of kindness, contributions to community or profession, talents, favorite jokes, oft-recounted experiences. When family
caregivers are exhausted, bereft, and possibly even ill, it is hard to remember those good times. Friends, relatives, and neighbors can help
to rebuild these precious memories.

CONSENT

I wait for death,
Not mine but Aila's.
How strange to wait for death
of another.
It puts a period on the sentence of life.
The very concept means acceptance,
And yet acceptance means consent.
Have I agreed to let her die?
I wait for death.
By what right have I agreed
to see it come?
Come it will, but must I consent?
Can I not reach out and hold her,
perhaps keep it at a distance,
to disperse its power with my presence.
I am indeed a fool to believe
that I can stay the last
pinpoint of ink upon the page.
An accident of motion could
make the pinpoint drop,
finish without consent the final line.

—Arthur Olson,
The Dying of the Light

I REMEMBER RECEIVING A PARCEL *and a letter from an associate of my father's who lived on the other side of Canada. In the parcel was a gallon can of maple syrup. The note said: "Your father did me a great favor once. This is a small gift to express the esteem with which I remember him." I never did learn more about this story but suddenly my father was there vividly in my mind, and for a while the burden of his loss was lifted.*

CELEBRATE AND LIVE
Dedicated to Moyra Jones

Celebrate the memories! That was what you, my mentor, said.
I do, I do—celebrating's easy!
I have such lovely thoughts of our togetherness
From before year one of our marriage until now—year fifty-three.
We've enjoyed each other in so many ways:
He taught me how to let go, to laugh, to play, to love
Even to cook, although he couldn't,
and I'd avoided that necessity.
So how can I easily give him up to Alzheimer's?
Memories are always fun to celebrate, but not alone!
Live the realities! That's tough and disciplined and real!
I've always been romantic and a dreamer;
This helps me to escape realities.
I still see my love as a dear and funny guy.
I need him to nourish me—
To help me with the pitfalls I find all too easily.
I need him to brighten up the world and love me.
I do not want to give him up
Although I know he's vanishing—piece by piece—
into Alzheimer's.

> —Gil Ludeman,
> *Journey into a Caring Heart*

Staff, too, have wonderful stories to tell. It is not unusual for professional caregivers to be welcomed into family circles; after all, they play an intimate role through all the stages of dementia. Staff members suffer bereavement too, repeatedly losing people they have grown to care for over many years. Sharing stories and memories helps everyone heal.

Once death has occurred, facilities who practice Gentlecare find many creative ways to celebrate the person who has gone. Some conduct memorial services, or wakes during which everyone exchanges stories about the person in order to celebrate his life. Some move the life panel or significant picture from the bedroom into a memorial hallway. Some burn a special lamp for 24 hours. More and more families dedicate living memorials to their loved ones; these may take the form of a therapeutic garden, a resource library, or a fund for dementia education or research. These important bequests enhance the life of a wide circle of people, and are a vital way to remember a loved one lost to Alzheimer's. One of the most effective and courageous memorials is created when family members volunteer their services and advocacy after their loved one has gone.

Of course, the best memorial of all is a healthy caregiver who is left with the strength to build a new life. This would be the wish of every person who has ever died of dementia. But recovery from caregiving is a long and difficult process, and it helps if caregivers don't have to experience it alone.

Do not stand at my grave and weep; I am not there. I do not sleep.
I am a thousand winds that blow. I am the diamond glints on snow.
I am the sunlight on ripened grain. I am the gentle autumn's rain.
When you waken in the morning's hush I am the swift uplifting rush
Of quiet birds in circled flight. I am the soft stars that shine at night.
Do not stand at my grave and cry: I am not there. I did not die.

—Mary Frye

DON'T LEAVE

Don't leave my love, not yet.
What will I do without you?
Who will share my thoughts?
Who will I laugh with?
Who will hold me and love me on
cold winter evenings when the windows
are iced and the sheets snow?
Who will share my dreams if you go?

Give me your hand.
Don't leave, not yet.
Don't leave.
Please!

> —Arthur Olson,
> *The Dying of the Light*

Time does not heal. It just pushes things into the
back of our consciousness. What heals is what we
do with time. Grieving heals. The way home is joy
through the heart of our pain. We have to grieve
until we come out the other side of it.

> —Deborah Duda,
> *Coming Home: A Guide to Dying*
> *at Home with Dignity*

Epilogue

Plus ça change,
plus c'est la même chose.
— Alphonse Karr, 1849

A great deal has changed in the years since dementing illness destroyed the lives of my father and mother. And yet far too much remains the same.

Earlier this year a woman phoned me in what can only be described as utter despair. Her story is only too familiar to those of us who advocate for people experiencing dementing illness, and their families.

Suzanne had been caring for her husband at home. At 61, he was in the throes of Alzheimer's disease. Although functioning well enough to attend a Victorian Order of Nurses day care program, Ted was becoming increasingly anxious and agitated. He was experiencing awful pressure to move around. This anxiety and restlessness resulted in his being unable to remain at rest long enough to eat, sleep, use the bathroom, or relax. This excessive need to walk and walk and walk was having a harmful effect on both his health and that of his wife.

Suzanne decided to seek help. With the aid of her family physician she admitted her husband to a specialized, government-sponsored program for dementia assessment and treatment. It was her hope that medical specialists could somehow relieve the pressure that was causing her husband to be so restless and uncomfortable.

The following events are described from *the family's perspective*. Of course, there are always two sides to a story. The family's story is told here because for too long this perspective has been ignored and not heard.

What follows is the way one family felt...was made to feel. This was the agony and uncertainty they experienced. This terror and impotence shaped their "days of hell."

DIRECTLY ON ADMISSION, *Ted was administered medication to reduce his anxiety. This medication was increased, discontinued, and other drugs were substituted. The family did not know which medication was given or in what quantity, since this information was never discussed with them.*

What they can describe are the changes they saw in their husband and father.

Ted quickly became frightened and hostile. He resisted staff's efforts to care for him. Most of the time he was comatose. Within days, despite or because of medication and physical restraint (depending on your perspective), he had become belligerent, pushing and hitting at staff and other patients. He was described to the family by staff as violent and dangerous. Although designated as an institution providing specialized assessment and treatment for dementia, the staff appeared at their wits' end to manage behaviors that Ted was now exhibiting.

Several days later, he was transferred to the psychiatric unit of the acute care hospital. The staff on the psychiatric unit described Ted as too aggressive to manage, and told the family that they "feared for their lives."

I'm not sure that it is possible for anyone who has not experienced it to imagine how devastating it is to hear a beloved member of your family described this way.

In such circumstances, a family caregiver is buffeted by emotions of anger, denial, shame, and guilt: anger that anyone could ever say such things; denial that a family member could behave in such a way;

Ted under the effects of medication.

shame that your family is being seen in such compromising public circumstances; and guilt...overwhelming, recriminating, energy sapping guilt, that you ever allowed such an experience to happen in the first place.

Suzanne thought:

- "Why did I ever complain about the behavior that was occurring at home?"
- "How could I have thought it was a problem compared to the mess we are in now?"
- "Are there other, better places I should have taken him?"
- "Are these the best doctors I could have engaged?"
- "Should I speak up more?"
- "Am I failing him?"
- "Are my actions going to result in his suffering and death?"

THESE THOUGHTS SWIRLED *through Suzanne's head as she prepared to attend a case conference to discuss Ted. She found herself alone in the conference with 11 professional staff. Although she had gone to the meeting prepared to present Ted's side of things, and armed with some resource materials she thought might help the staff, she was soon overwhelmed. She describes how even her normal gumption and good sense drained away, leaving her uncertain and vulnerable.*

The psychiatrist who presided at the conference explained that they planned to move Ted to another hospital, since the present location did not have the proper environment. This was very evident to Suzanne, but also puzzling, since the unit he was in was specifically designed as an assessment and treatment resource center.

The psychiatrist informed Suzanne that it had been necessary to invoke the Mental Health Act and have Ted certified as mentally incompetent. This action was not discussed in advance with the family, though at least one member of the family had been with Ted every day; nor were the implications explained.

Suzanne's power of attorney was swept aside with this legal manoeuver. She was to learn later that only a specifically convened review panel could examine an appeal on her part. And this action enabled the staff to apply four-way restraint to Ted and to confine him to a darkened room.

Suzanne now saw her husband in a darkened room, physically restrained hand and foot, nearly comatose with medication, and virtually unable to eat or drink.

What had she done?

How could this be happening?

Where could she turn for help?

At this point, Suzanne was approached by a care attendant who told her about a workshop she had attended where the Gentlecare system of dementia care had been presented as an alternative approach. Suzanne called me. I advised her that, working with her physician, she must quickly find alternate care for Ted. I suggested she visit a privately owned, specialized dementia care facility that had a few government-sponsored beds. Here she would find specially trained staff, a dementia-specific environment, and appropriate care strategies and programs. Because the facility used the Gentlecare model I also knew that no physical or chemical restraints would be used. I further provided her with information regarding a few legal advocates that work on behalf of people's rights within the health care and mental health systems.

Suzanne knew the moment she stepped inside the door of the facility that practiced Gentlecare that this was the place for Ted. Here he could move about freely through spacious indoor rooms and a beautiful outdoor park. Here the staff were not afraid, but interested and supportive. They understood how Ted was feeling; they felt his pain and confusion and appreciated how difficult life was becoming for him.

Most importantly, here they knew how to build a prosthesis to compensate for his dysfunction. Here was a physician who could monitor Ted's care over time in conjunction with family and staff. And signifi-

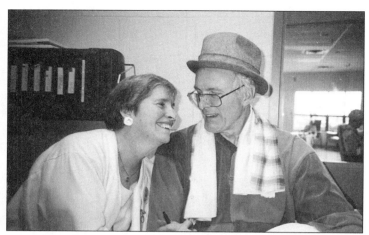

Ted with staff member: the joy of having someone you can count on.

cantly, here Suzanne had found a haven for her family. This was a place where her feelings were important, her knowledge critical to Ted's care, and her presence vital to his very life. Within a few short miles, she had gone, in her own words, from "hell to heaven."

TED'S PHYSICAL CONDITION CHANGED *quickly and dramatically. And most surprising of all, his cognitive ability began to return. Within a day he was walking with help, and was soon out in the garden with his wife. He began to bond with and trust staff members who were able to assist him with all his activities of daily living. All of us began to enjoy Ted's courtly manner and funny conversations. Slowly his life returned to normal—normal for someone experiencing dementia.*

Ted's family moved from a place of darkness to a place of hope, from impotence to empowerment. They clearly see a possible quality of life for both Ted and themselves as this horrific disease plays out its course. Suzanne's own health has moved away from the brink of illness as the burden of stress is relieved.

Nothing makes Alzheimer's disease OK. But knowing that your afflicted family member is comfortable and supported in his attempts to manage life activities is a help. So does having staff members who respect the family's position and listen to them. Knowing that you can move ahead with your own life without sacrificing your health and happiness helps too. All of these factors make it possible for family caregivers to join with professional staff in a creative partnership of caring to support people living with dementia.

How many Suzannes and Teds must there be before we stop replaying this costly scenario? When will health care planners understand that the biomedical model just doesn't work for people with dementing illnesses? When will our physicians and psychiatrists become aware of alternatives to the biomedical model, which work miracles for people with progressive dementia—over and over and over again?

Is the fact that almost no research into care strategies is being undertaken the reason for lack of support for alternative approaches?

We are not documenting the staggering costs incurred when our health care system turns people like Ted into totally dysfunctional individuals, and turns family caregivers into new consumers of health services because their own health breaks down. Families are simply too weary and frightened to search out different care.

Those of us who advocate for people experiencing Alzheimer's disease or other dementias can only believe that the chaos swirling around dementia care will eventually evolve into humane and effective ways of responding to the needs of these vulnerable people.

Places like the haven that Ted and Suzanne found must replace the highly technological acute care approach that utterly destroys families living with dementia.

They cost less.

They work.

But isn't it time we began to really help victims of dementia? After all, who are these people?

Who am I?

You may wonder.

I am someone you know very well.

For I am every man you meet.

I am every woman.

I am you.

Ted and Suzanne enjoy a daily walk in the garden of the facility where he now lives.

(This is a true and recent story. Only the participants' names have been changed. Ted now lives in a lovely facility in the Lower Mainland of British Columbia, Canada, visited regularly by his wife and family.)

Index

(Italicized page numbers refer to illustrations)